In Which
Winnie-the-Pooh
Protects the Hundred Acre Wood
from Eczema

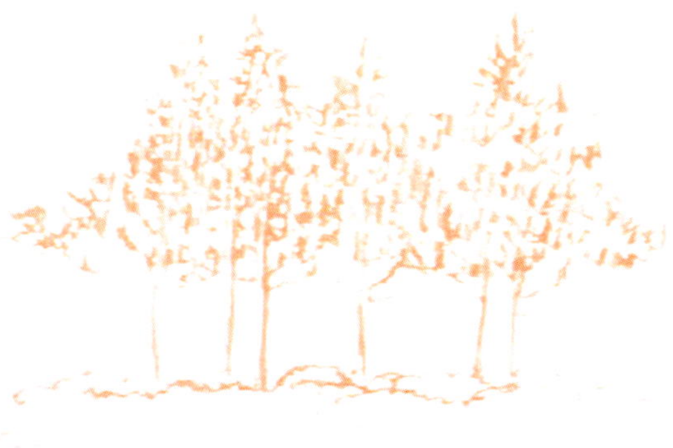

Drs. Ian Myles & Nadia Bhandari

Illustrated by
Nadia Bhandari

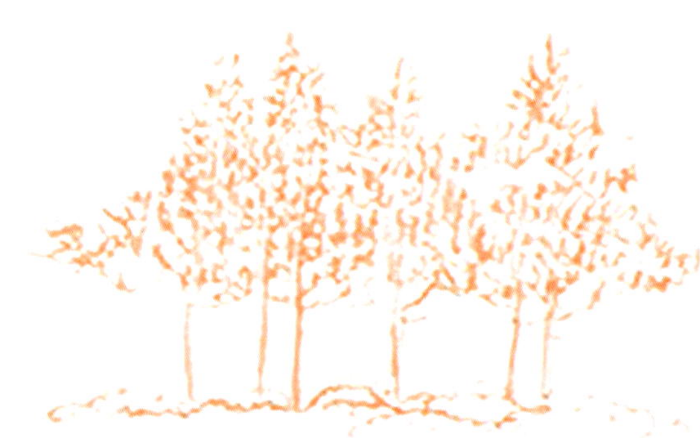

ISBN 979-8-9892309-4-5

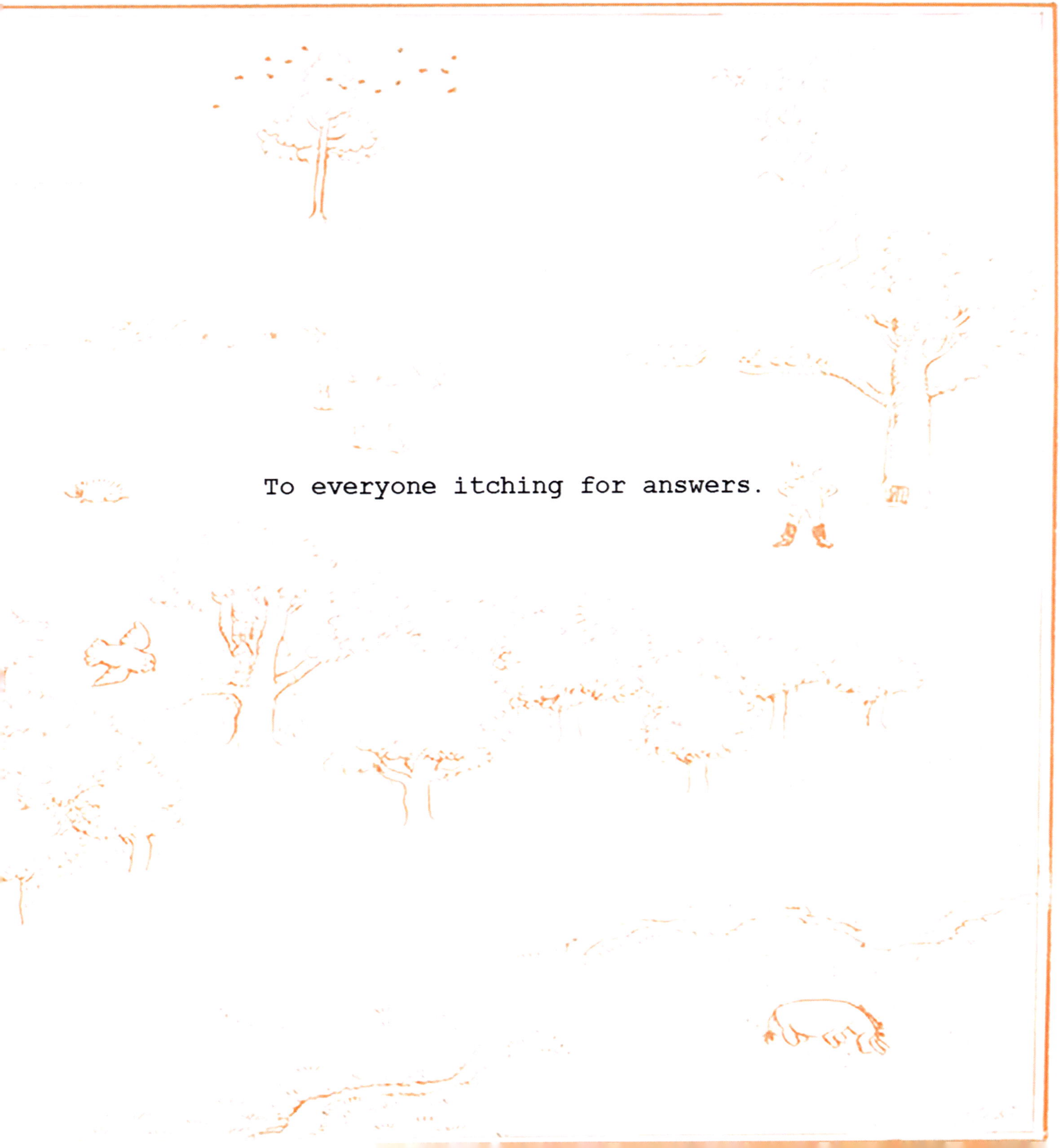

To everyone itching for answers.

It was a bright and sunny day
in the Hundred Acre Wood, so
Pooh and Piglet went to visit
Christopher Robin.

But Christopher Robin was
still in bed.

"Hello Christopher Robin,
would you like to come out and
play today?" asked Pooh.

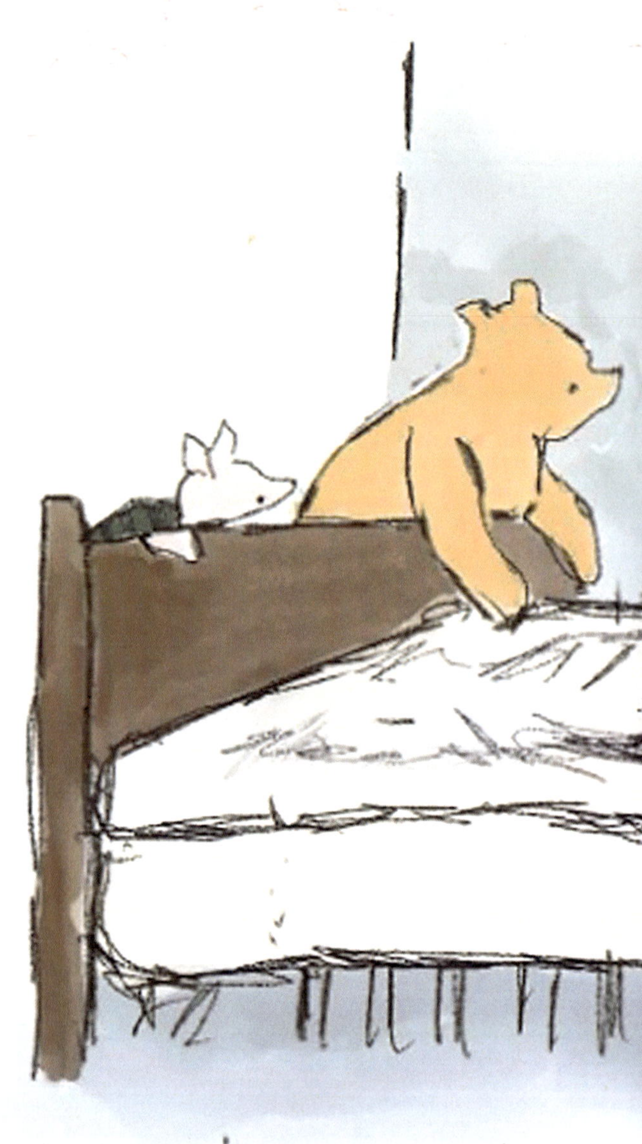

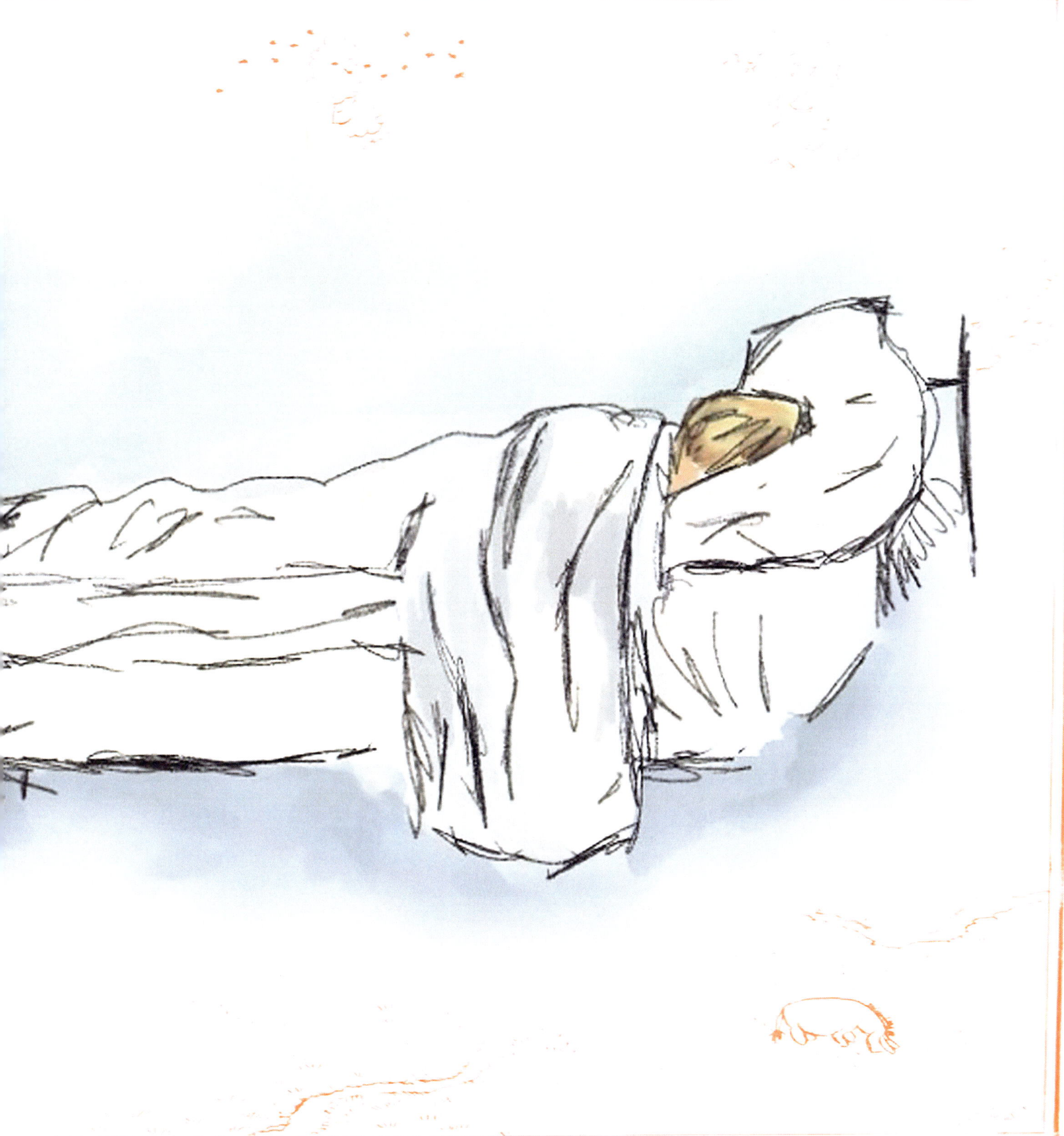

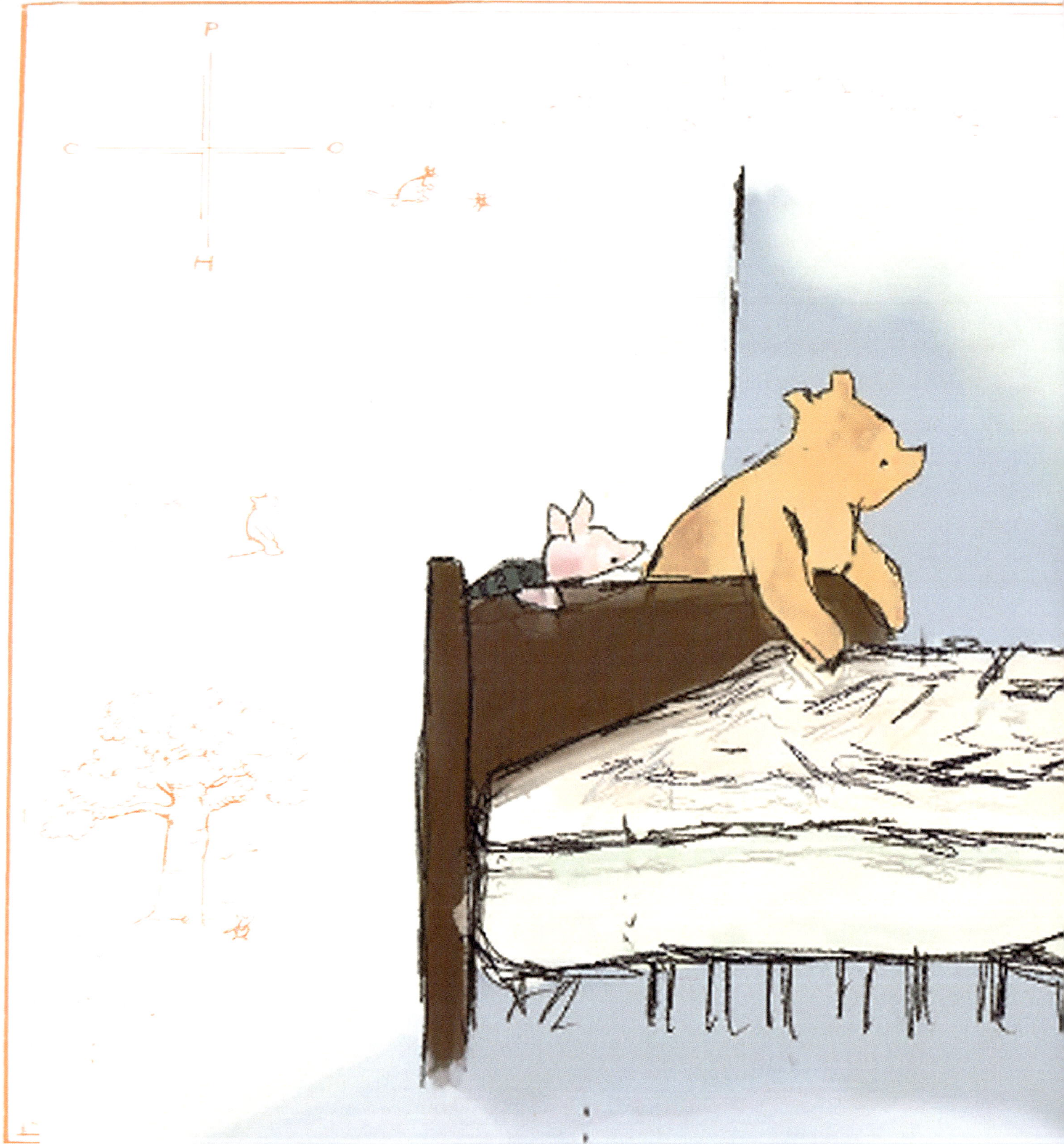

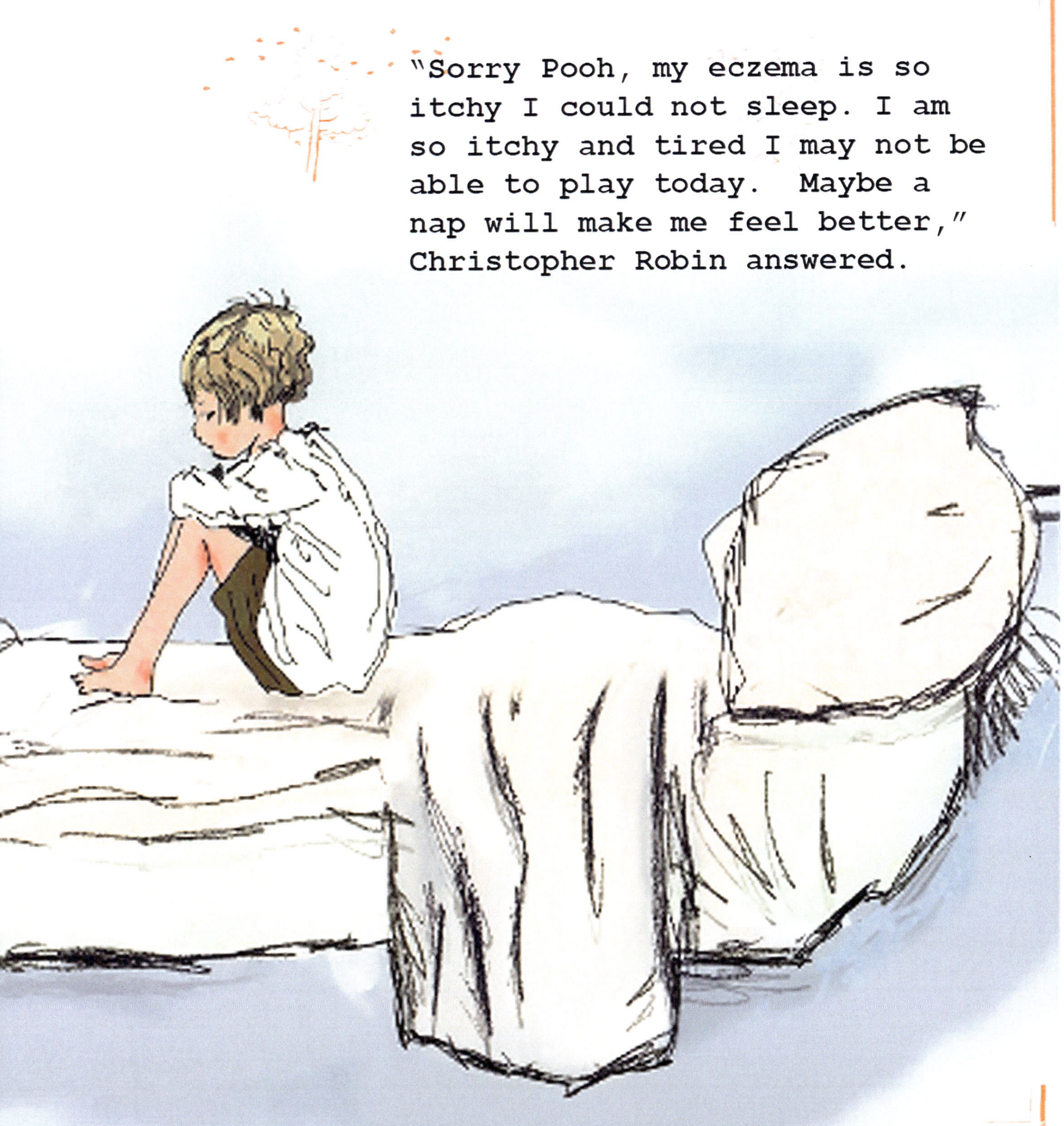
"Sorry Pooh, my eczema is so itchy I could not sleep. I am so itchy and tired I may not be able to play today. Maybe a nap will make me feel better," Christopher Robin answered.

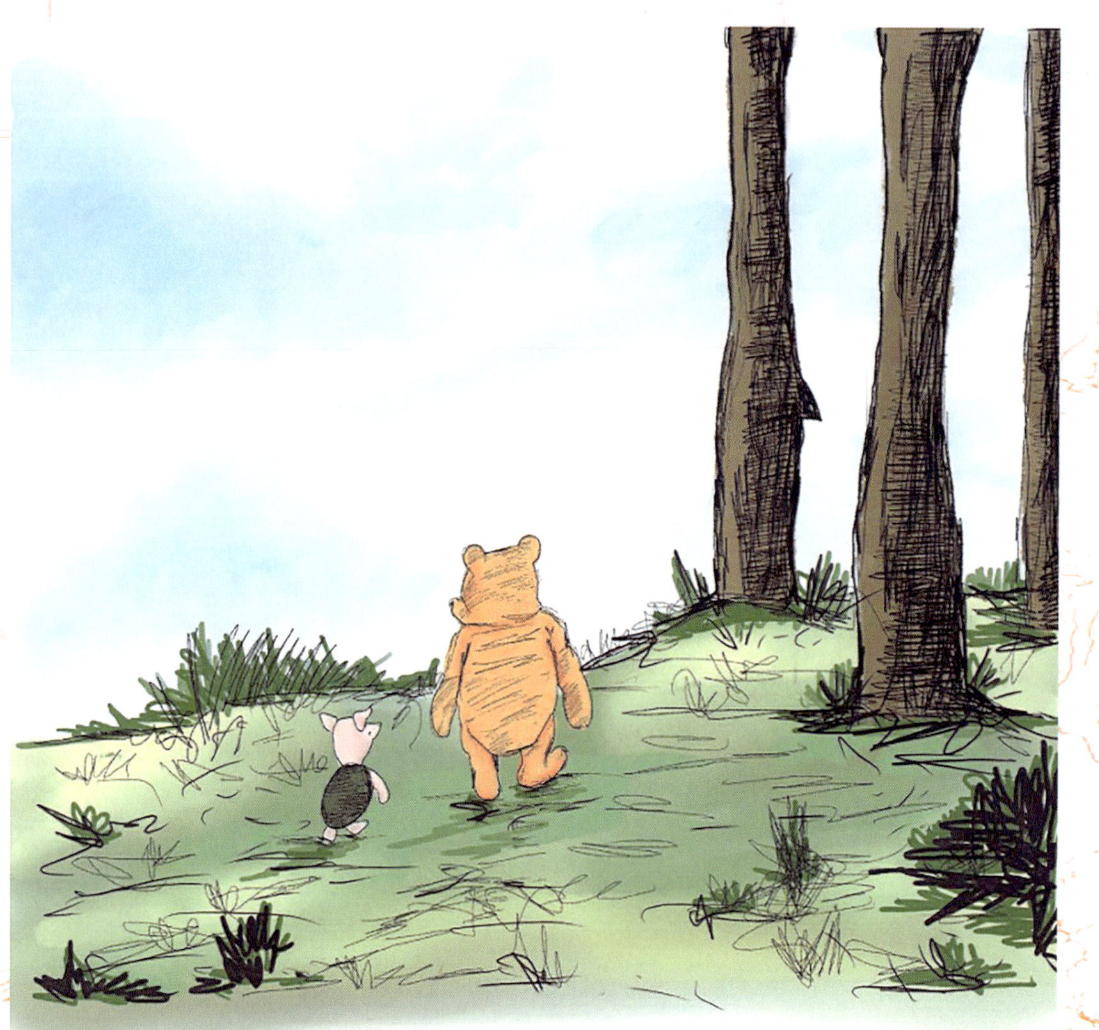

Pooh and Piglet left Christopher Robin to
sleep. They started walking back to Pooh's
corner.

"Oh, pah-pah-poor Christopher Robin,"
Piglet said.

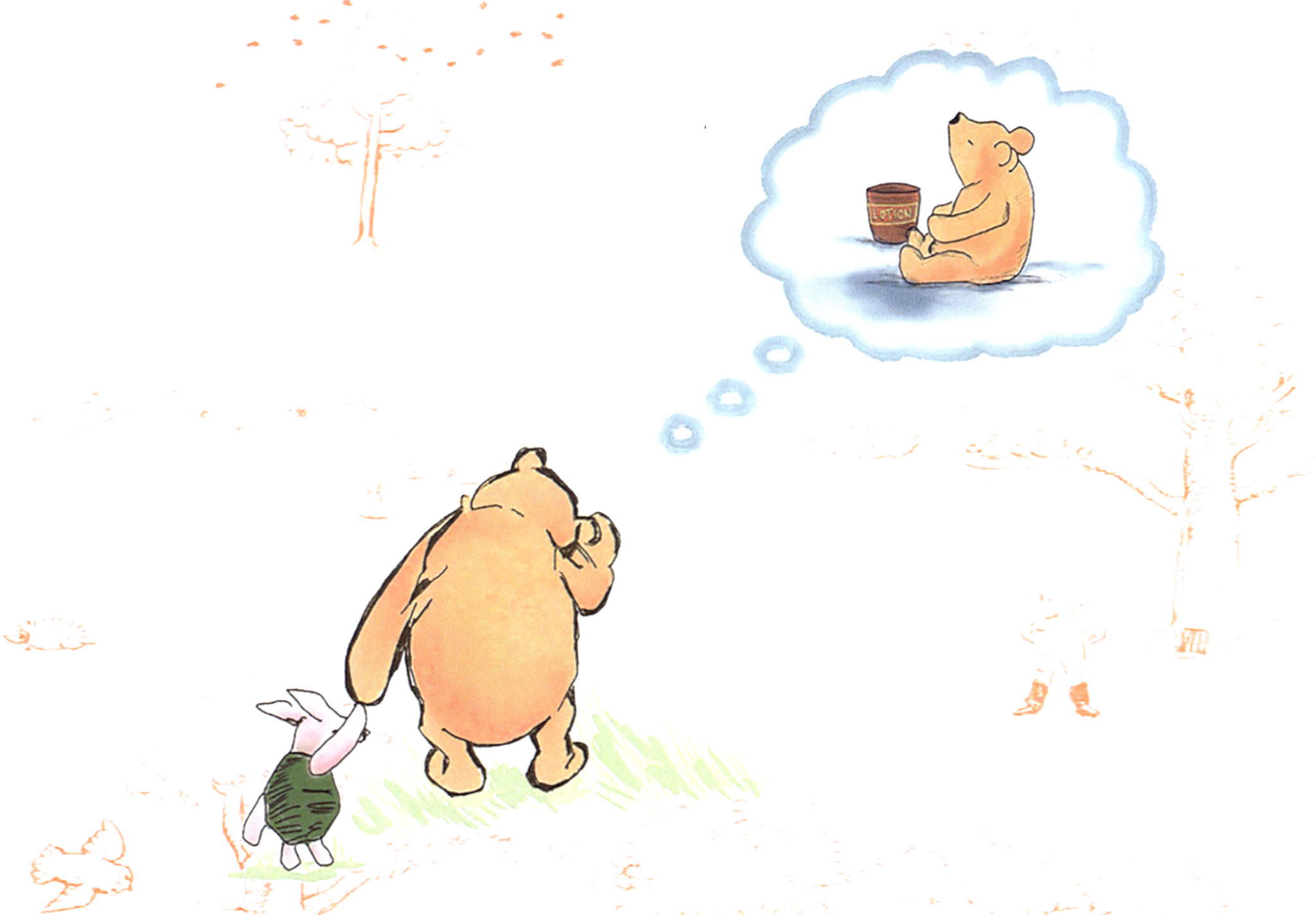

Pooh felt sad for his friend and started thinking
about ways he could help. "I think I might have
a jar of something that could help in my house.
Owl said it was good for 'zema since it has no
woozle powder in it!" Pooh said.

"Are there other things that might help 'zema?"
asked Piglet.

"I think so, Piglet. Let's go ask Owl if he knows
what else we can do," said Pooh.

While walking towards Owl's house, Pooh and Piglet came upon Eeyore floating in the stream.

"Hello Eeyore," said Pooh.

"Hi, Pooh. Hi, Piglet," Eeyore groaned.

"What are you doing in the water, Eeyore?" Piglet asked.

Eeyore replied, "Just my luck, my eczema has flared today and the itch is too much. I am soaking so my skin won't feel so dry."

"Sorry Eeyore," said Pooh. "You know, Christopher Robin is also having a 'zema flare. There must be something in the Hundred Acre Wood today. We will tell him that a bath can help!"

"Yes, I suppose the bath might help," Eeyore said gloomily as he watched Pooh and Piglet continue down the path to Owl's house.

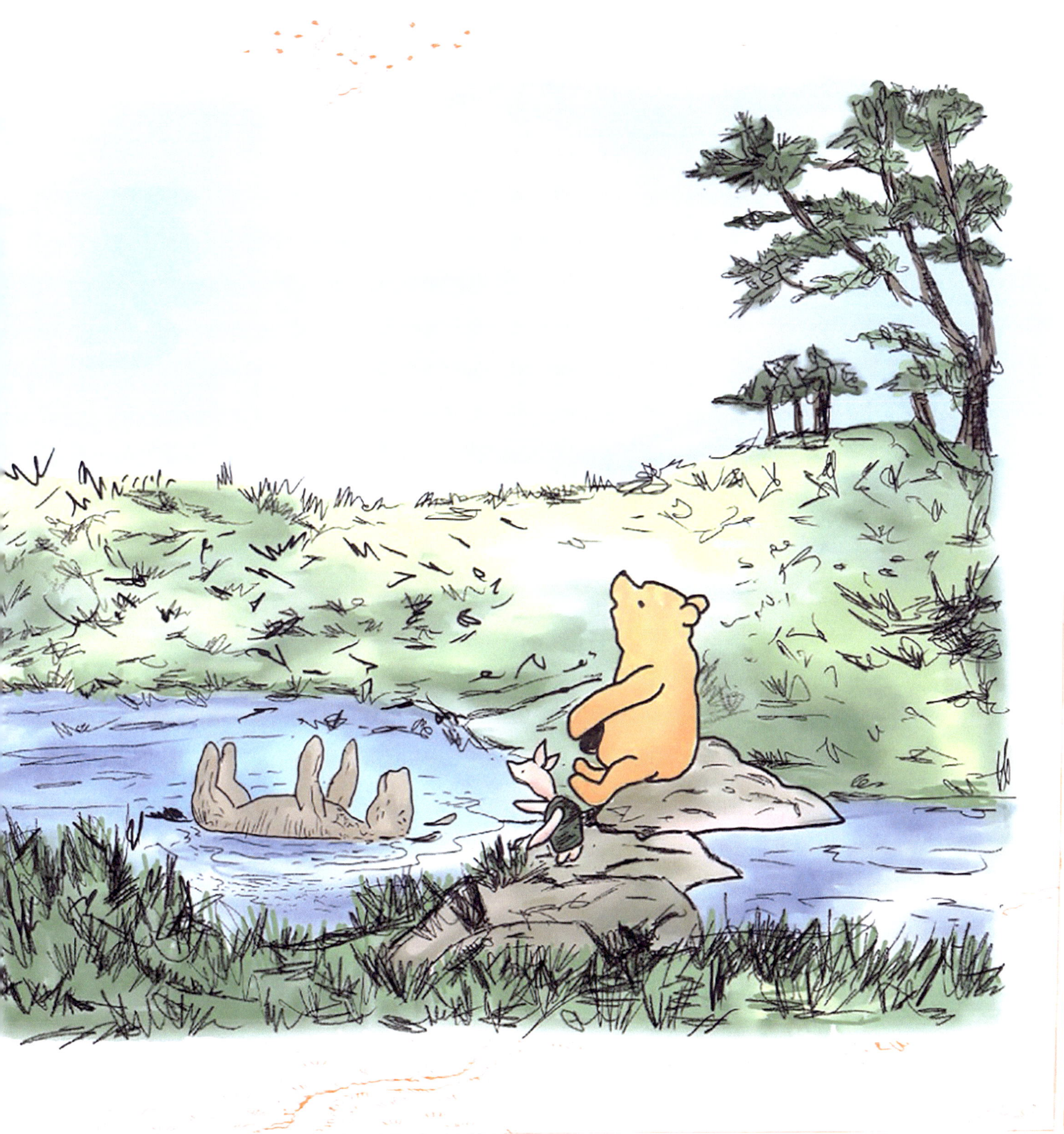

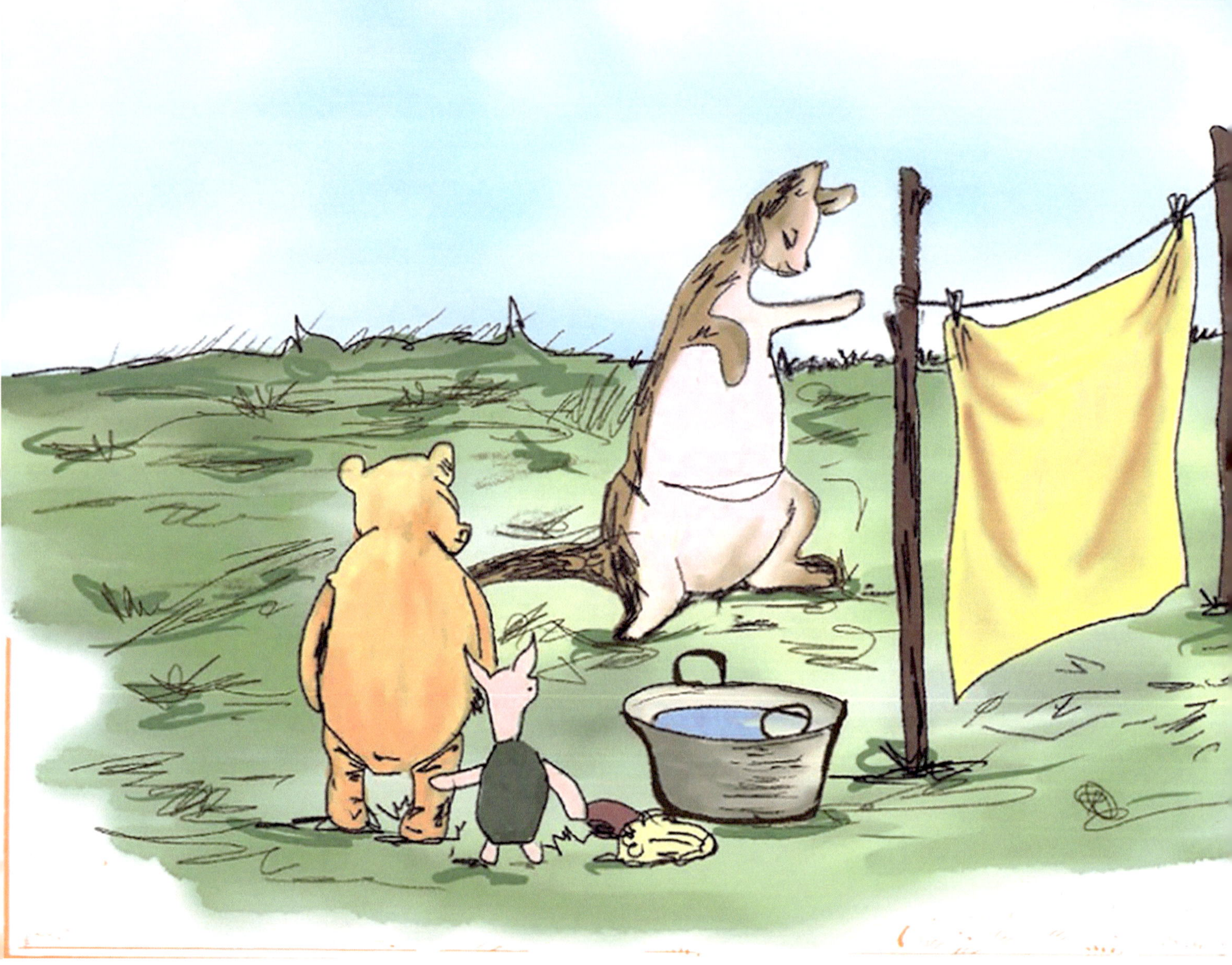

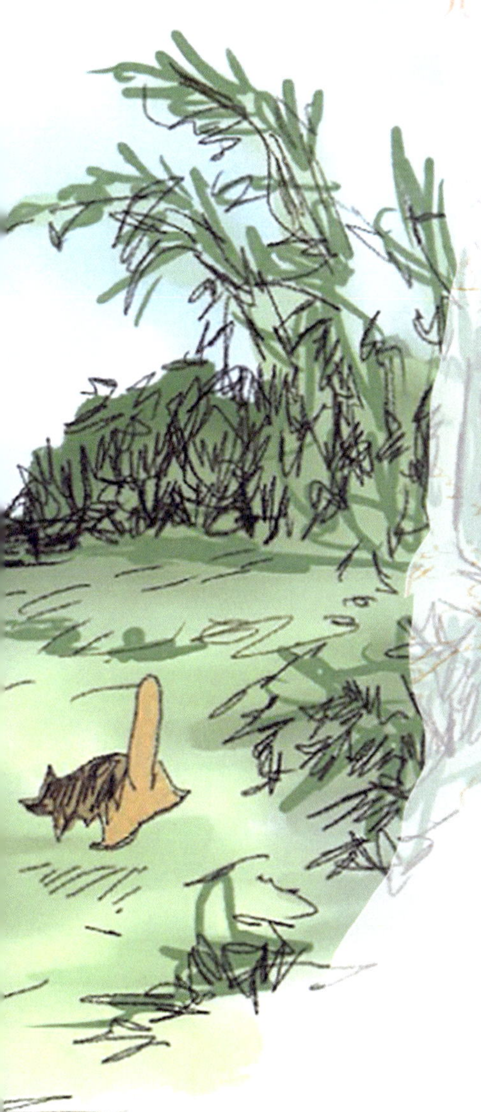

As Pooh and Piglet crossed the field, they saw Kanga outside with Roo. "Hello Kanga, how do you do?" Pooh said.

"Oh hello Pooh. Where are you going today?" Kanga asked.

"We are headed to Owl's house to ask how we can help Christopher Robin's 'zema" Piglet replied.

"Ah yes, I heard everyone's eczema is bad today," said Kanga, "I'm washing his blanket with special soap. When you have eczema, you have to make sure your soap does not have any heffalumps!"

"Thank you, Kanga. When we talk to Owl, we will be sure to tell him the good news about Christopher Robin's blanket not having heffalumps anymore," said Pooh.

As they were walking towards Owl's house, Pooh and Piglet suddenly heard a strange buzzing sound. "What's that noise, Pooh?" Piglet asked in a scared voice. "Are those ba-ba-ba-bees?!"

"Oh bother, those would be the strangest sounding bees I've ever heard," Pooh replied, "The buzzing seems to be coming from Rabbit's house."

"Rabbit, are you home?" Pooh shouted as he stuck his head into Rabbit's window.

"AH! Pooh, you startled me!" Rabbit said in a huff.

"We were headed to Owl's to help Christopher Robin's bad 'zema day but heard some strange buzzing. Do you perhaps have bees in here, or maybe just some honey?" Pooh asked.

"No Pooh, that is my air cleaner. It gets all the bad air out of my house," Rabbit said.

"Would this air bee machine help 'zema?" Pooh asked, scratching his head.

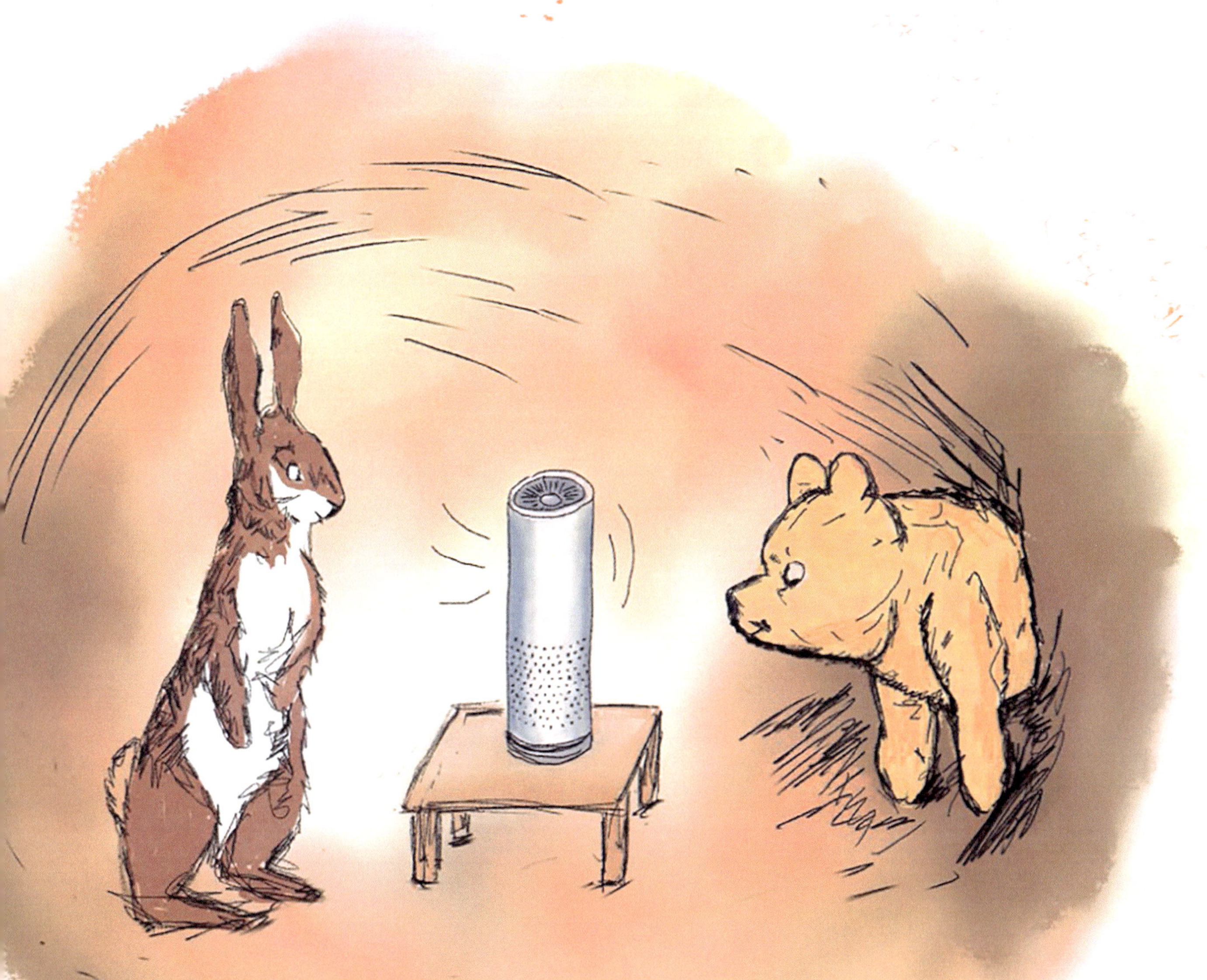

"Yes," Rabbit replied. "On blustery days, I can clean the air coming into my house by opening a window and putting up a filter. But today, I need an air cleaner. I use it a lot, especially if someone with eczema is visiting!"

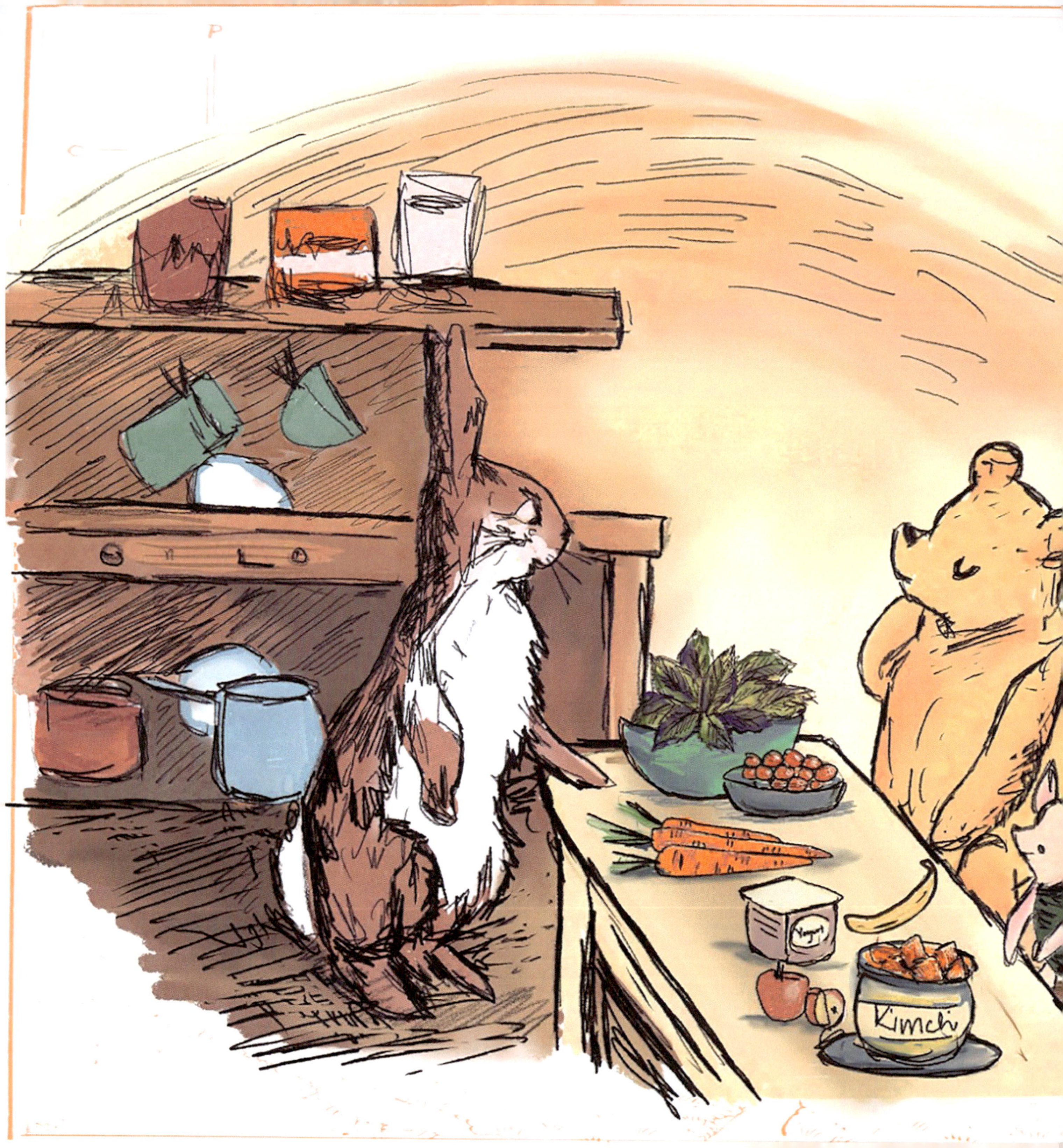

Kimchi

Pooh nodded thoughtfully but started to feel a sensation in his belly. All this talking about 'zema had made him forget about eating. Then, Pooh noticed some yummy food on Rabbit's table. "What have you got there, Rabbit?" asked Pooh
.

"Well, I am visiting Christopher Robin for lunch, so I am bringing veggies, fruits, yogurt, and kimchi for him. Owl says when you have eczema, you have to eat fresh foods and foods with probiotics," Rabbit said.

"What are pah-pah-probiotics?" Piglet asked.

"They are tiny little helpers in some special foods, like kimchi or yogurt. They are so small you can't see them. But they live in your tummy and help keep you healthy," Rabbit explained.

"I think I feel my little tummy friends rumbling for something yummy. Do you perhaps need help tasting a bit of this food, Rabbit?" Pooh asked.

Rabbit shared some crunchy carrots. With a full belly, Pooh and Piglet started back on their way to Owl's house.

Knock, knock knock!

Owl opened the door, surprised to see his friends.

"Hello Owl," said Pooh and Piglet.

"Hello Pooh and Piglet. I'm just getting ready to go visit Christopher Robin. What brings you here?" asked Owl.

"Christopher Robin's 'zema is making him very itchy and sad. Do you know how we can help him?" Pooh asked hopefully.

"Why yes, Pooh! I was just headed to his house to make sure his room does not have any heffalumps or woozles around," Owl said. "I can teach you about all the other things we can do on the way there."

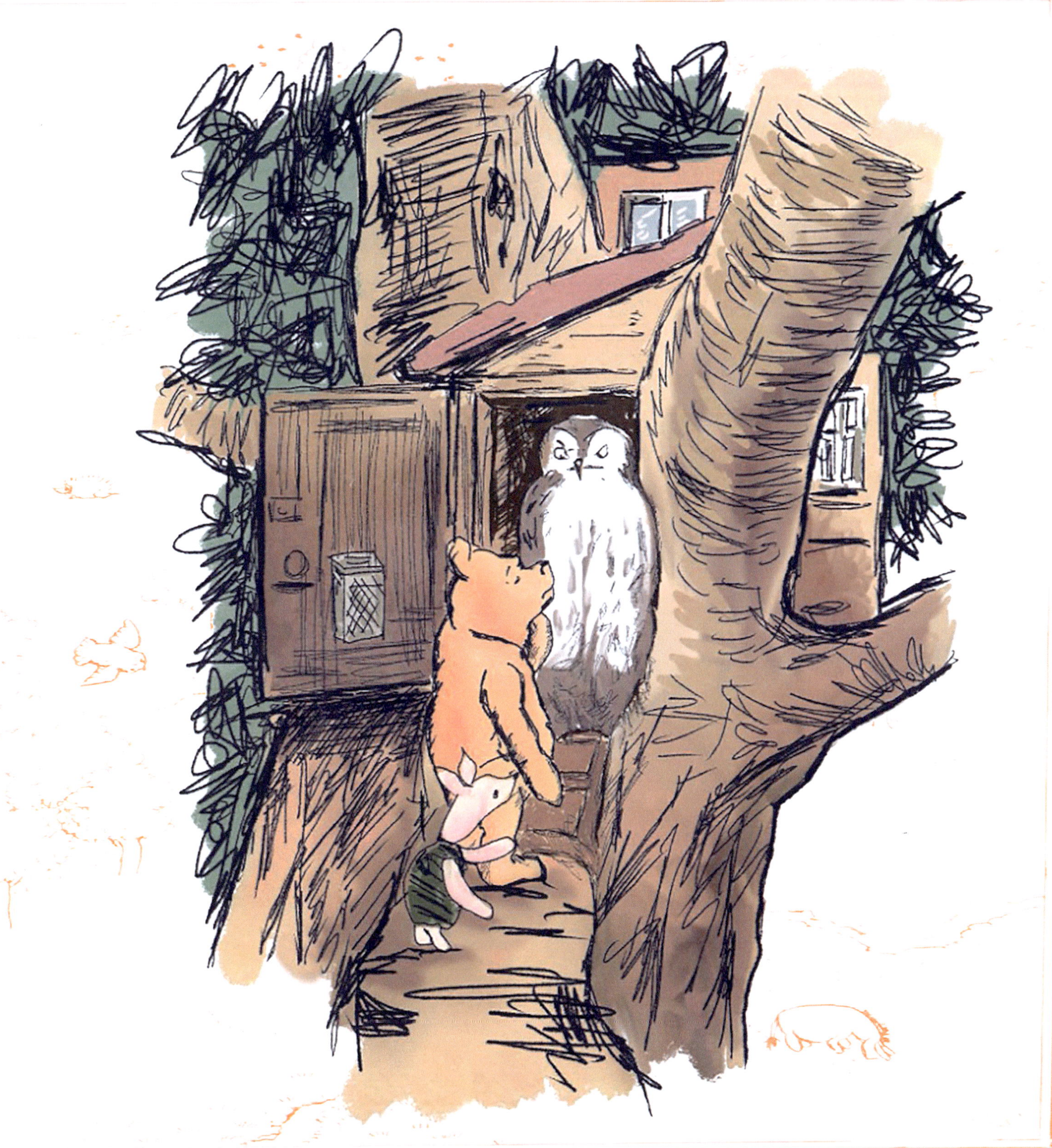

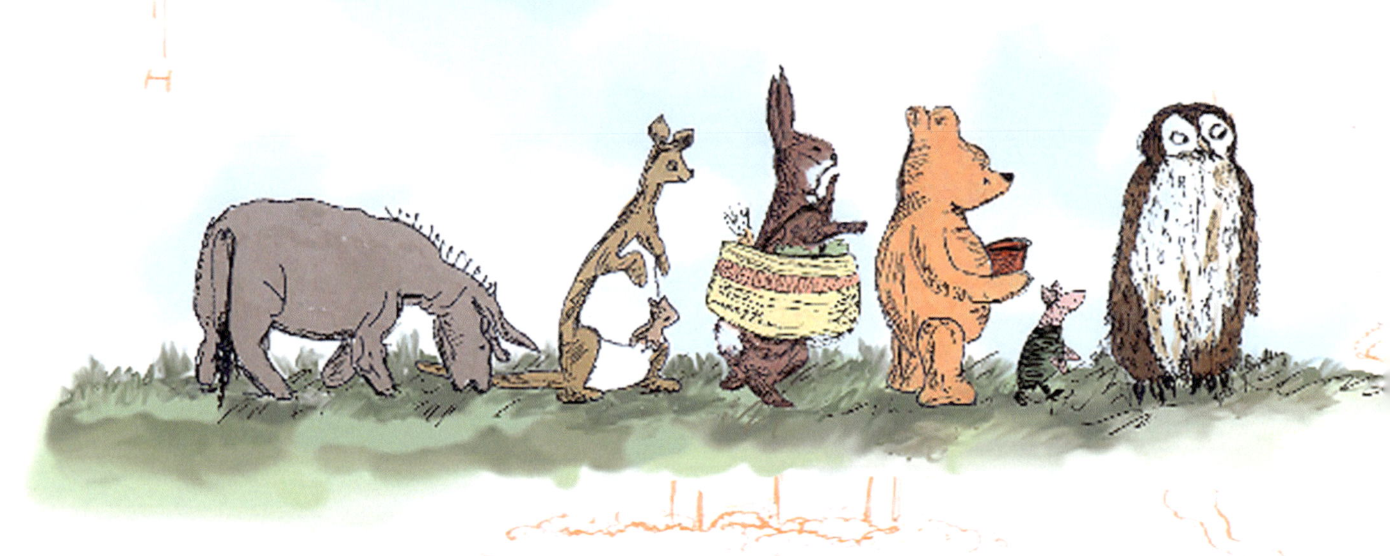

So Pooh, Piglet, and Owl walked back through the Hundred Acre Wood. They met up with Rabbit, who brought a basket of yummy fresh food and the air cleaner. Kanga and Roo joined next, carrying a clean blanket for Christopher Robin. Pooh stopped by his house to grab his woozle-free lotion… and a quick taste of honey. They all talked Eeyore into joining them now that his bath was done.

While everyone prepared for lunch, Pooh walked
into Christopher Robin's room and told him about
everything he had learned about 'zema.
Christopher Robin decided to take a nice
soothing bath while he listened to Pooh and
Piglet talk about the day's adventures.

Christopher Robin then put on the special lotion
right after getting out of the bath, so his skin
wouldn't feel as dry and itchy. "Wow Pooh, this
lotion really helps, thank you!" he said.

"You should use it at least twice a day if your
skin feels dry," Piglet said with a smile.

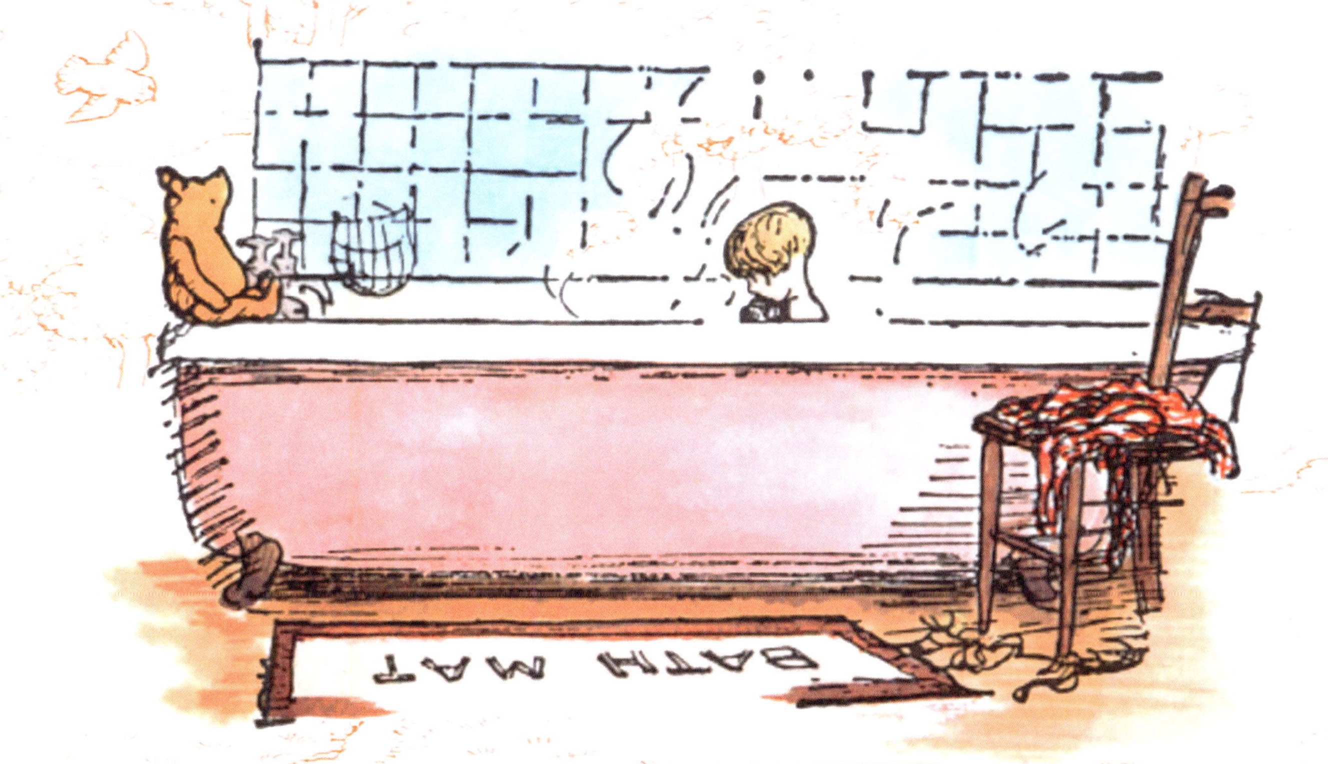

After his bath, Christopher Robin
decided to come outside to visit
everyone for a picnic lunch.

"Christopher Robin, how are you
feeling with your eczema?" asked
Owl.

"I feel a bit better now,
especially since you all are here
to help. Thank you for this clean
blanket, Kanga, and these yummies,
Rabbit." Christopher Robin smiled.

After lunch, everyone helped clear
all the heffalumps and woozles out
of Christopher Robin's room.

"The most helpful thing when you
have eczema," said Christopher
Robin, "is to have friends and
family that care about you!"

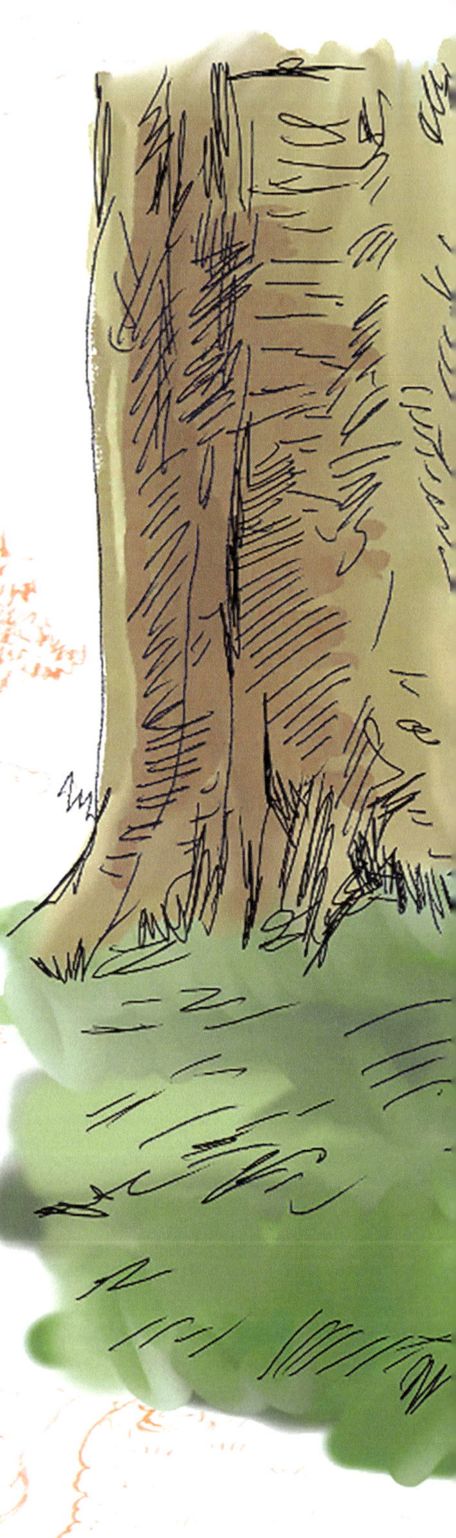

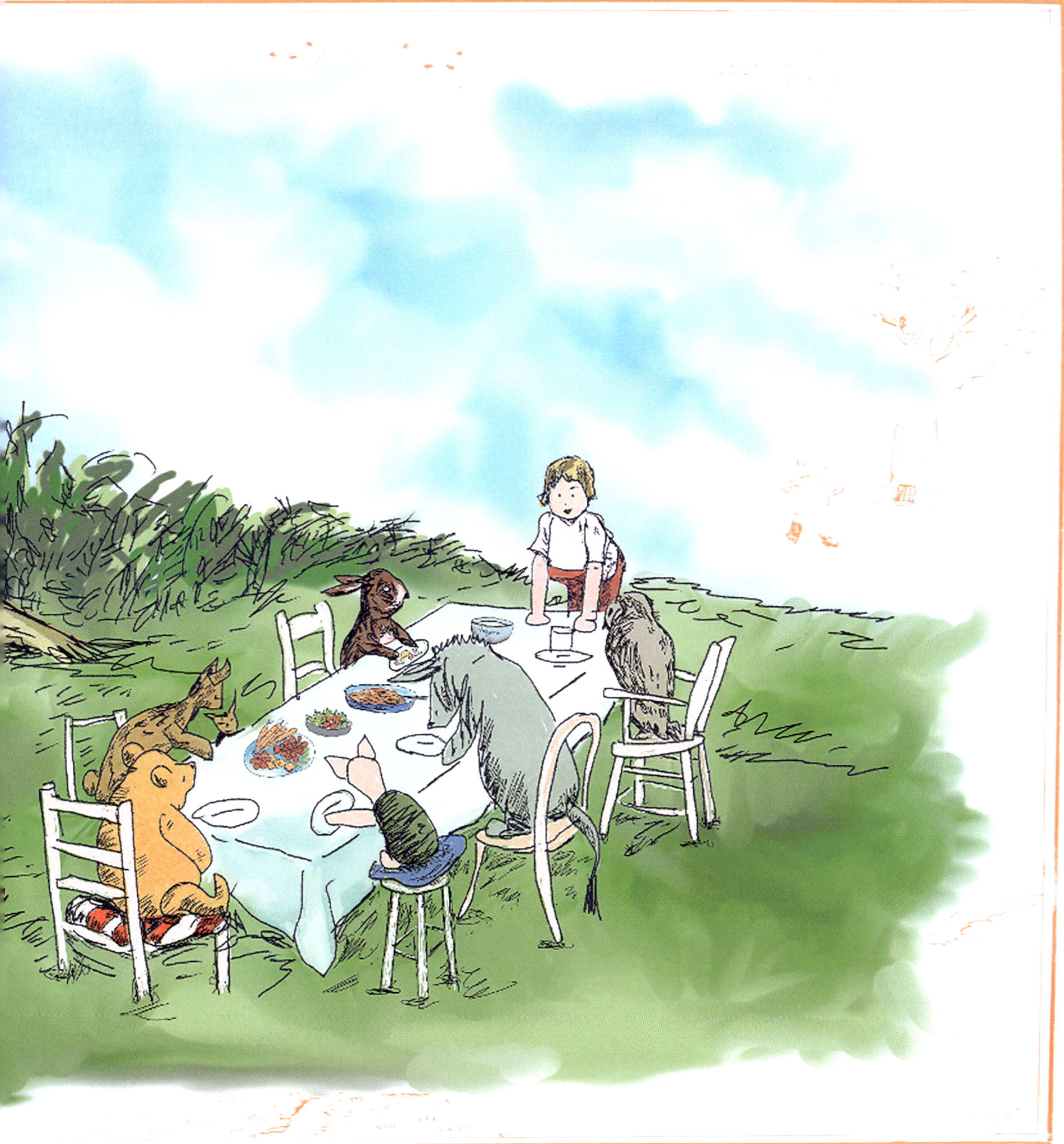

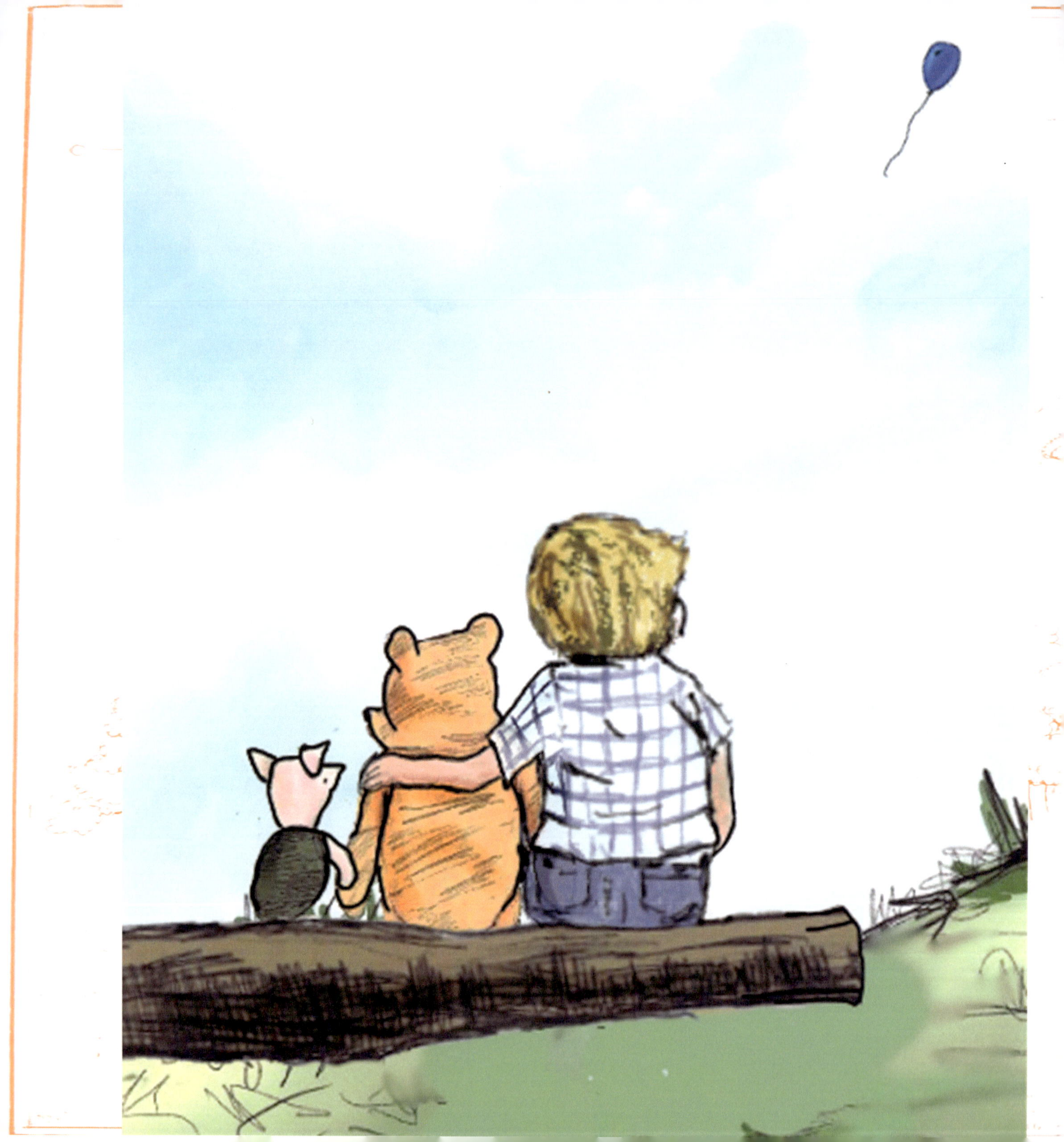

Christopher Robin, Pooh, and Piglet sat on
their favorite log and thought about everything
they learned that day. Piglet felt less
worried now. Pooh was not so bothered but was
still a little hungry for some more honey and
carrots. Christopher Robin was feeling better
and hoped the work they did would help keep his
eczema away. But even if his eczema returns,
he would still have his friends.

THE END

PARENT PAGES

This section is meant for parents to help detail ways Pooh and friends helped remove things that may have worsened Christopher Robin's eczema. But first, we should set expectations. We expect that changing your environment will lower the rate of flares and help control your symptoms. Even if these changes don't completely cure your child, there is good evidence that they will help. So please talk to your health care provider about any medications you have been given to see how what you are currently doing to control your eczema fits in with this advice.

Things to think about inside the home:

When selecting products for the house such as bedding, cleaning products, and detergents, try to avoid products with chemicals* that might worsen eczema. In the book, we referred to these products as containing "heffalumps". Examples include volatile organic compounds (usually abbreviated as VOCs), formaldehyde, isocyanates, and more. These can be difficult to avoid, since many products won't tell you if these chemicals are used as ingredients.

----

* Technically the term is "toxicant," but we will
  use the term "chemical" for simplicity.

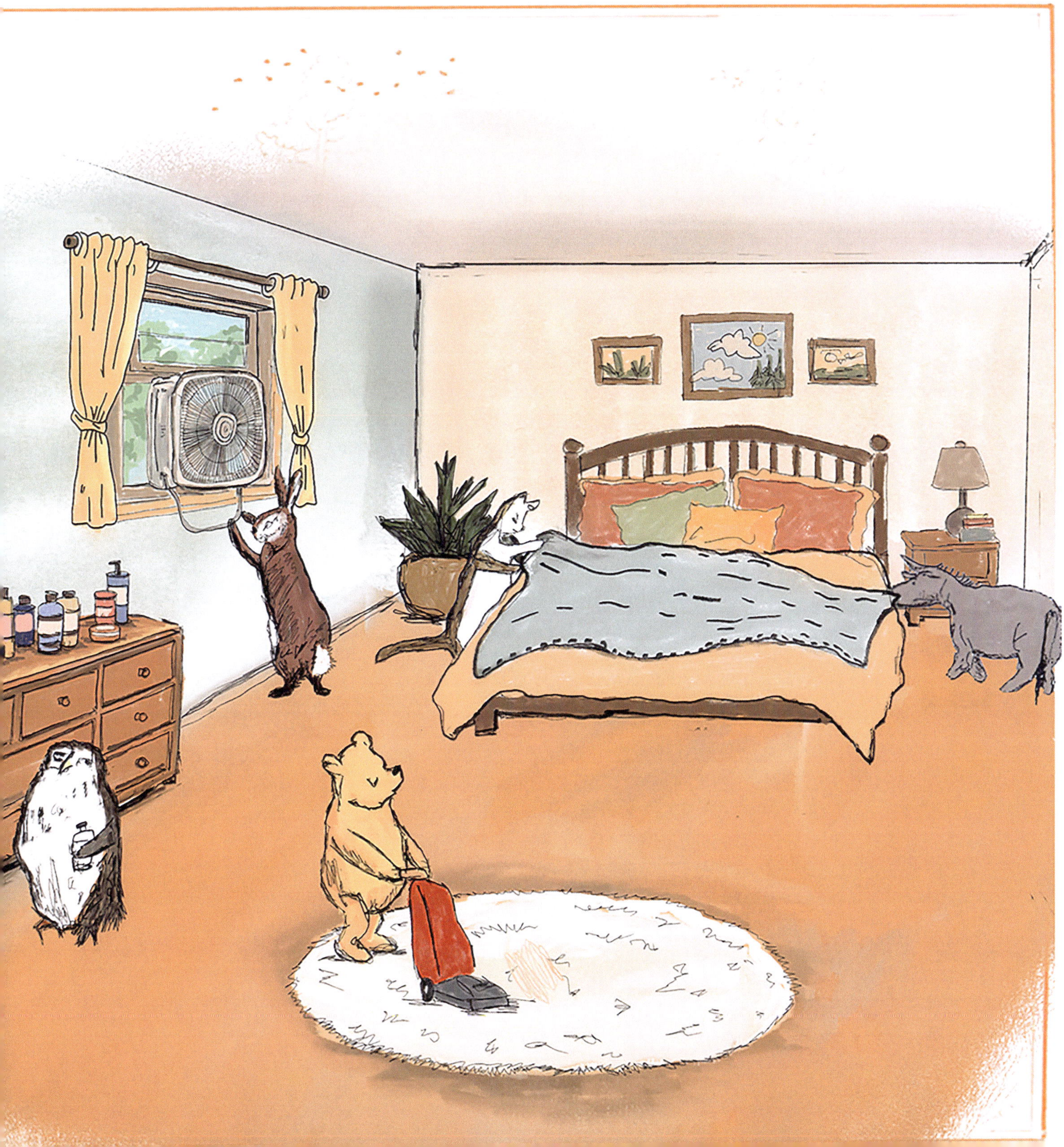

Parents can use phone apps such as Yuka (1), EWG's Healthy Living (2), SkinSafe (3), or Trueview. These apps allow you to scan the bar code on the packaging and, if that product is in their database, the app will report what chemical harms you should worry about. Other options include the Allergy & Asthma Friendly program from the Asthma and Allergy Foundation of American (AAFA, more info at aafa.org/certified). The AAFA program certifies products as free from chemicals that may be harmful for patients with allergies, asthma, or eczema. The AAFA certifications even include guidance on things used in home renovations like insulation, paint, and flooring. The list isn't perfect, but it is a great start. That said, the risk of eczema is significantly greater in kids if their bedroom or nursery is renovated before the age of four years (4-6). This is due to the increased risk of chemical exposure from things like new wallpaper, paint, flooring, and more. Unless there is a structural need, remodeling a newborn's nursery for purely aesthetic reasons is something you might consider avoiding until at least six years of age.

Other ways these chemicals can sneak into your home is through toothpaste and cooking supplies. Check your toothpaste to make sure it does not contain something called sodium lauryl sulfate (or SLS) (7-8). SLS harms the function of the gut lining and is linked with allergic diseases. Also, teflon pans contain chemicals known as PFAS. While these chemicals are not as strongly linked to eczema (9), they are implicated in asthma.

Please note that when a product is labeled "green," there is no
assurance that it is free from eczema-causing ingredients.
Some studies suggest "green" products may contain lower amounts
of harmful chemicals than other products (on average), but you
cannot use the label "green" as a guide for avoiding any
specific chemical (10). Like toothpaste, try to avoid laundry
detergent with SLS. You should also avoid products that are
marketed as improving the shine on glassware (like rinse aid or
others)(11). The chemical used to shine the glasses also
erodes the function of the gut lining and is linked with
allergies. Again, the apps mentioned can be used to confirm
whether products contain these harmful chemicals, or you can
look at the AAFA list for ideas.

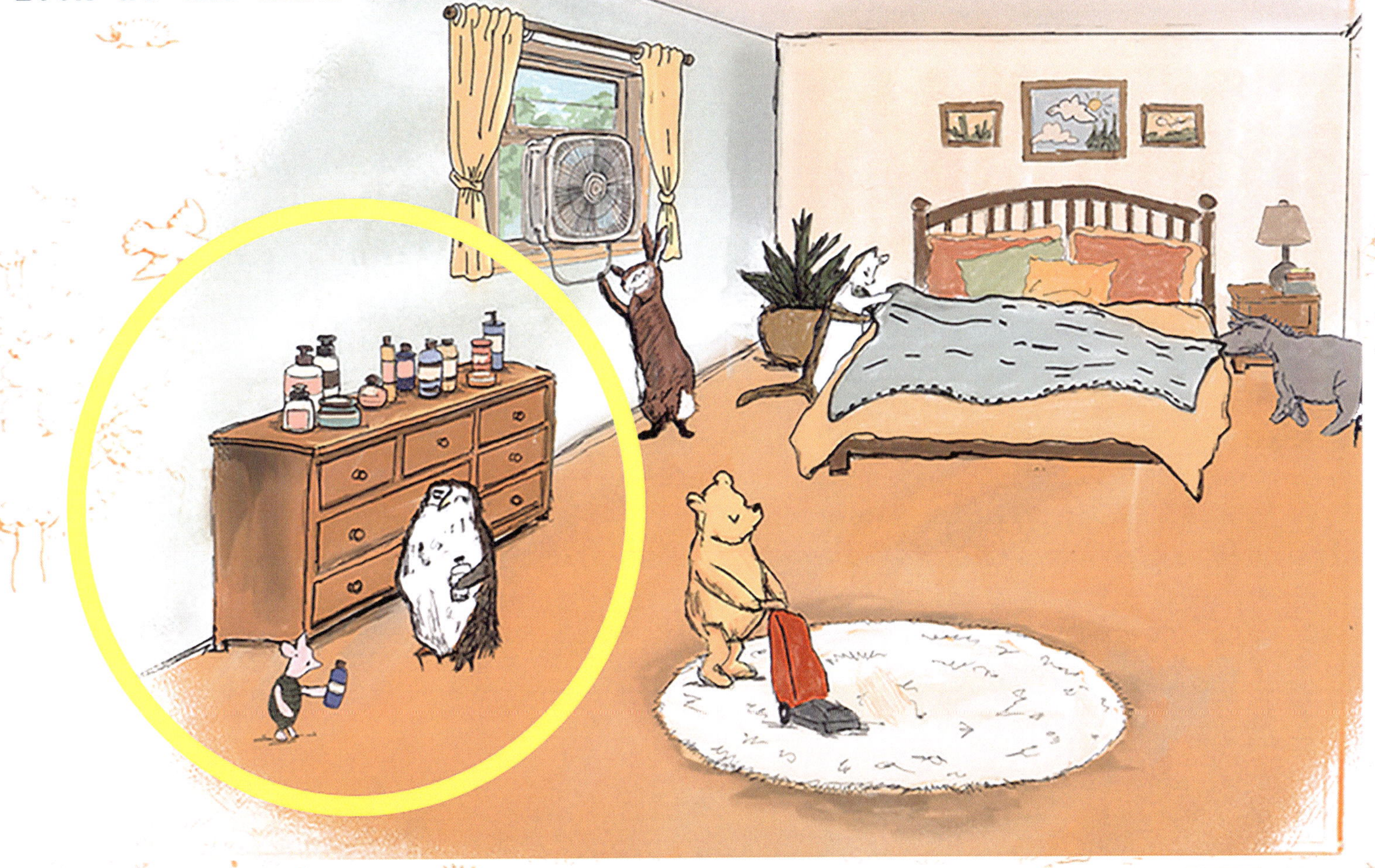

Bedding

Sleepwear (like pajamas and onesies) and bedding (sheets, blankets, and pillowcases) should be made of natural fabrics like cotton (12-13). While bamboo is a natural fiber, the production of bamboo sheets and clothing carries a risk of contamination that is not present for cotton (14-15). You may also consider that some child sleepwear is coated with flame retardants. Obviously, these have good intentions of reducing flammability, but there is evidence suggesting concerns that flame retardants - particularly on products pressed against the skin for long periods of time - might cause or worsen eczema. Any company selling the products should disclose the use of these coatings. For fabrics specifically, you can look up brands and products on the OEKO-TEX Standard 100 website. They certify products free of 100 different chemicals of concern (https://www.oeko-tex-.com/en/our-standards/oeko-tex-standard-100/).

In general, "memory foam" pillows and mattresses should be avoided, since they are often made with isocyanates (16-17). Beds made with latex foam are more likely to be safe. However, people with latex allergies would only have cotton mattresses as options.

Related to bedtime, be mindful that a lot of stuffed toys are made with isocyanates or other VOC-emitting foams, particularly the inexpensive ones. Polyester and nylon, for example, are common - but both are made from chemicals that are known to worsen eczema (12-13). It is difficult to identify which ones have VOCs, but you should be able to look up if the contents are foam or cotton.

Even when made of cotton, stuffed animals and pillows can
harbor dust mites. There are plenty of "dust mite" pillow and
mattress cover options - but again, keep in mind many are made
of polyester and thus would not be the optimal choice. One
trick for stuffed animals is to put the toy in a plastic bag,
and then in the freezer overnight. That will kill the dust
mites without ruining the toy.

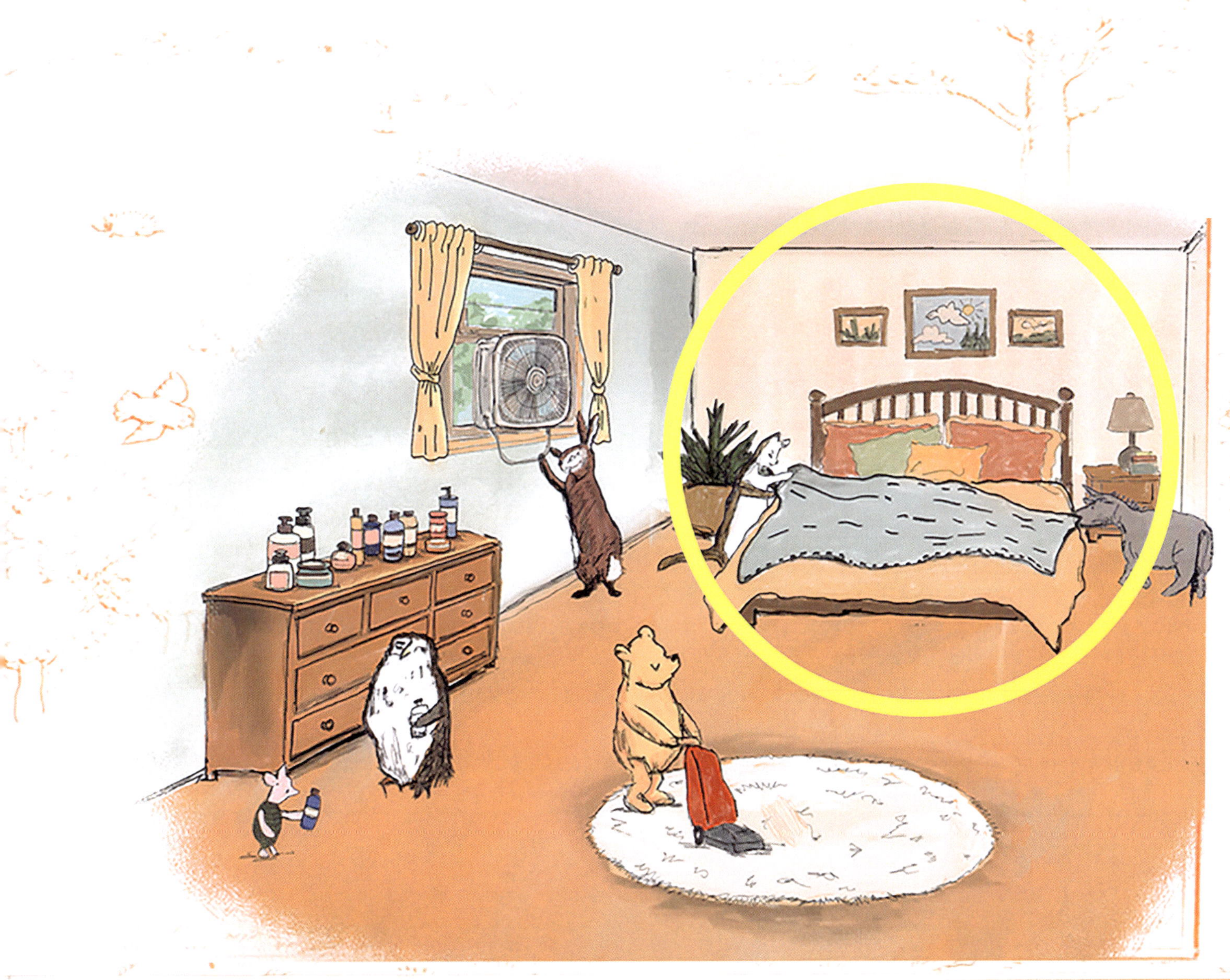

Purification and ventilation

Purification

Air pollution - from wildfires, cars, factories, and even products in your home - can worsen eczema. Two approaches are purification and ventilation - both are important (18). If you are shopping for an air purifier, make sure to get one that helps against VOCs. HEPA filters are the most common type but are aimed at catching dust particles, not VOCs. Filters against VOCs are usually made of "activated carbon." Thus, you should look for a filter with both a HEPA and activated carbon filter. Unfortunately, the AAFA currently certifies filters based only on their ability to remove pollen, not VOCs. Filtering pollen is still important, especially if you have hay fever. But, for eczema, the goal should be reducing VOC exposure. The last recommendation for filters is to assure that they do not produce ozone. Filters that claim to electrify the air or provide "chemical reactions" as part of their cleaning process might produce ozone. If your air purifier produces ozone, it is just replacing one type of pollution with another.

Three brands we like - and have no conflict of interest with - are: Rabbit Air (so long as you use the insert with activated carbon), Nuwave OxyPure, and Austin Air.

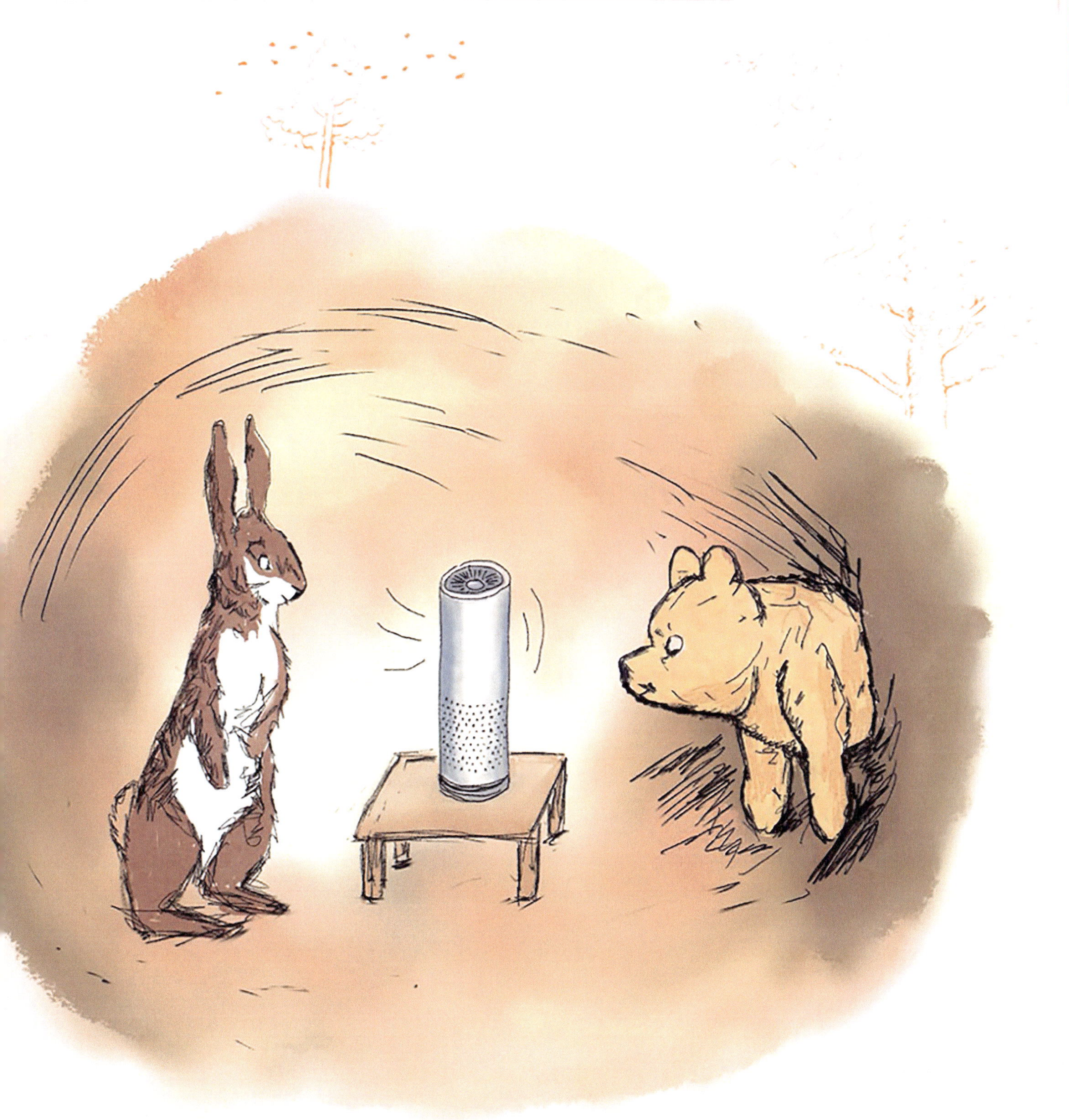

Ventilation

Ventilating your house is much cheaper than using air purifiers. It can be done with two box fans and one filter that is normally used in a home furnace. Here is what to do:
• Pick a window in your home/apartment that is closest to (or facing) the nearest major road.
• Put one box fan in the window facing out, so the air is blowing from your home out towards that street.
• Take the second box fan and tape a MERV 8 or MERV 12 filter to the front of it, so the air has to blow through the filter.
• Make sure the tape covers all of the sides of the filter, so air has to pass through the filter and can't sneak around the sides. Using filters with ratings higher than MERV 12 won't work as well because the fan won't have the power needed to blow air through it - so using MERV 12 should be fine. Here is an example of what the filter could look like taped to the intake fan:

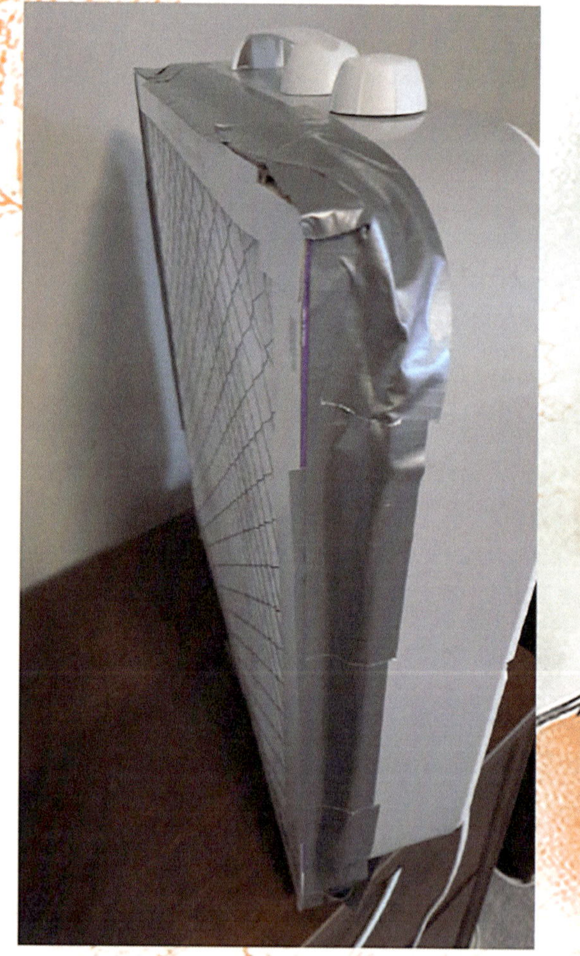

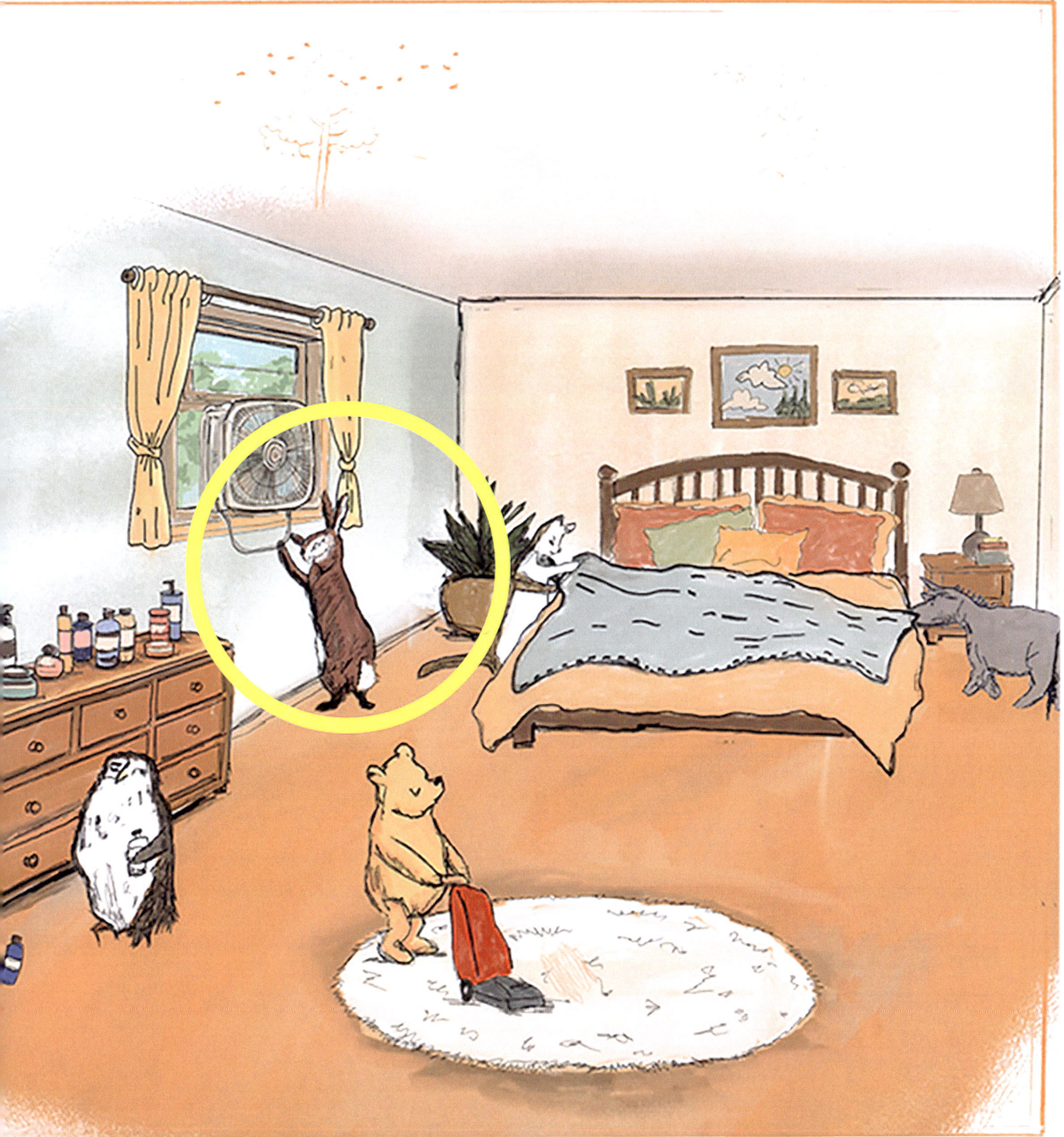

• Pick a second window, ideally one far away from, or facing away from, the closest major road. Put the filtered box fan in the second window facing inward.

With this setup, you will be pulling air in from outside and filtering out the pollens, dust, and particulate matter. Meanwhile, the other fan will be pushing polluted air out. Here are some pictures of an example setup:

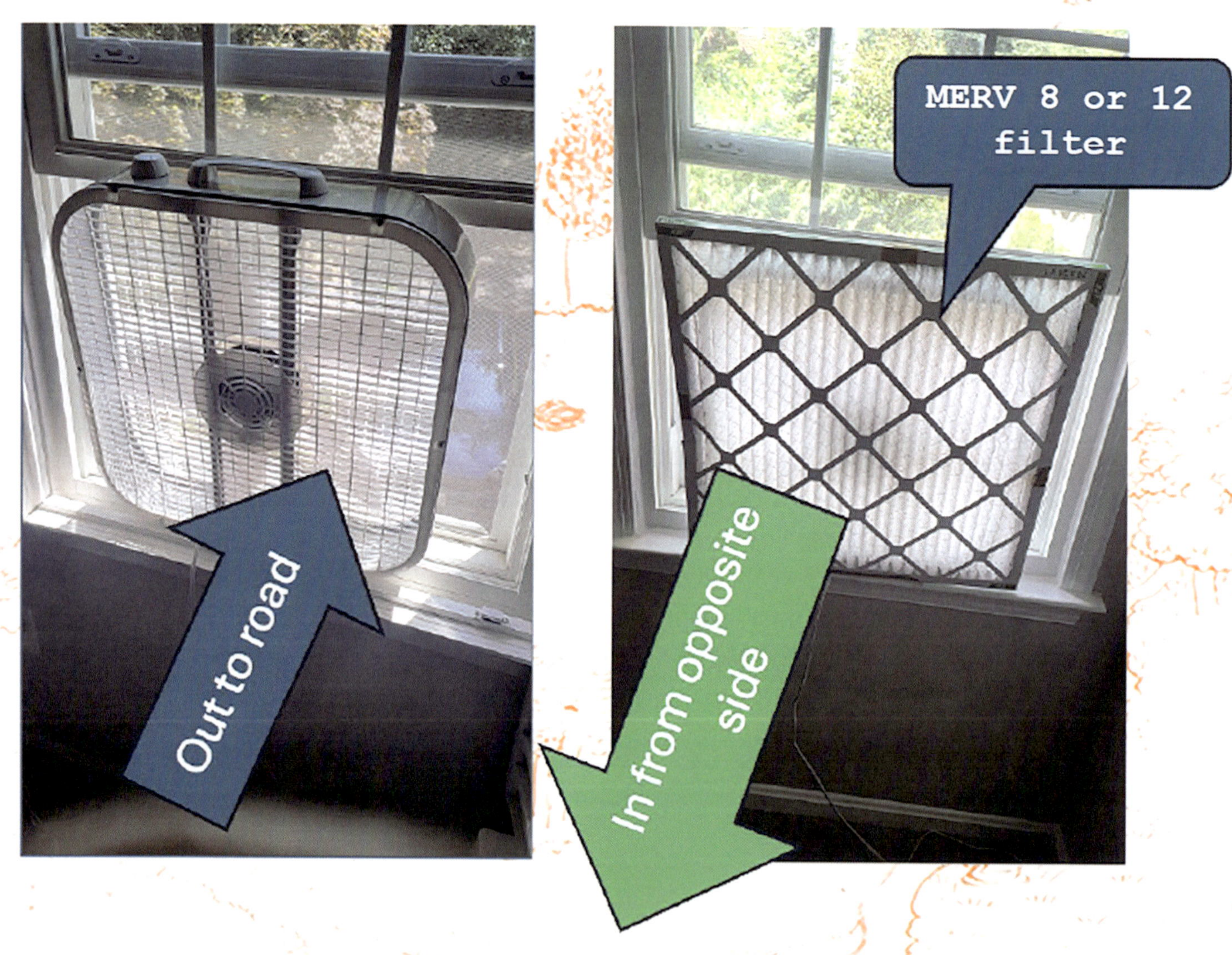

It is okay if the fan does not completely fill the window. The overall result will be to reduce the amount of VOCs and other harmful chemicals in your air. Numerous studies show that these chemicals concentrate indoors - so simply keeping the windows closed can actually be bad, because it might cause the chemicals to become "trapped" indoors (19-22).

Remember that both purifiers and the filters on the box fans become clogged over time. They should be changed at least every three months or maybe more, depending on the specific brand of purifier or how often you ventilate.

Remember to look through the products you use in the home to see if any give off VOCs using apps like Yuka and the others mentioned. When you vacuum, make sure to either run the air purifier or ventilate the house, since the vacuuming kicks up dust and particulate matter that might worsen eczema. Washing sheets and pillowcases frequently can reduce the amount of particulate matter and pollen that lands on the bed (so long as the detergent you use is free of heffalumps 🙂). You should also avoid candles or air fresheners in the home. All are designed to emit fragrances and other chemicals, which can be irritating to the skin of patients with eczema.

Finally, there are specific species of plants that have been shown to "eat" these harmful chemicals. Putting them in your home won't replace the need for ventilation or purifiers, but they can help and only require some water and sunlight. The specific species include: Areca palm, spider plant, golden pothos, gerbera daisy, boston fern, weeping fig, peace lily, chrysanthemum, snake plant, and/or aloe vera (23-26).

Diet

As frustrating as it is to admit, not much is known about what diets are best for people with eczema. What little scientific information is out there suggests eating fruit, vegetables, fermented foods (yogurt, kimchi, kombucha, fermented rice flour, kefir - fermented milk)(27-31), as well as what are loosely called "healthy fats" (which include chicken, fish, oats, brown rice, walnuts, sunflower seeds, avocados, lentils, and sweet potatoes). It is important to avoid refined or processed sugars and refined/processed fats. Sugar and fat in their more natural form are often complex when viewed by what specific molecules are being eaten.   When sugars and fats are eaten in their natural state (like sugar in fruit, or fat in nuts, meat, or fish), that can be healthy because there are lots of different types of sugars and fats being consumed. But when sugars and fats are "refined" or "processed," that usually means only one or two types are being consumed (32-33).

For example, apples have "sugar" (fructose) but also have fiber and other nutrients that make the whole apple healthy. But stripping away everything except the fructose makes that fructose something that can worsen inflammation. Same goes for fats - plenty of foods have saturated fats naturally. However, fat in processed foods is typically only one or two specific molecules (known as palmitic acid and stearic acid). These two specific molecules of saturated fats also induce inflammation, even though foods that contain them in a mixture with other types of saturated fats can be healthy. Often, foods with high processed fats also have emulsifiers which help keep the fat mixed in with the rest of the product. Examples include lecithin, xanthan or guar gums, or polysorbates.

An unfortunate side effect of emulsifiers is that they disrupt
the cells in the gut and can cause inflammation. These should
be consumed in moderation.

We have provided a visual representation of what an "eczema
food pyramid" might look like - except not a pyramid since we
don't know which of these healthy foods should be put on top.
It is meant as a guide to help understand which foods have
evidence supporting the idea that they help with eczema, even
if that evidence is not as great as we would hope.

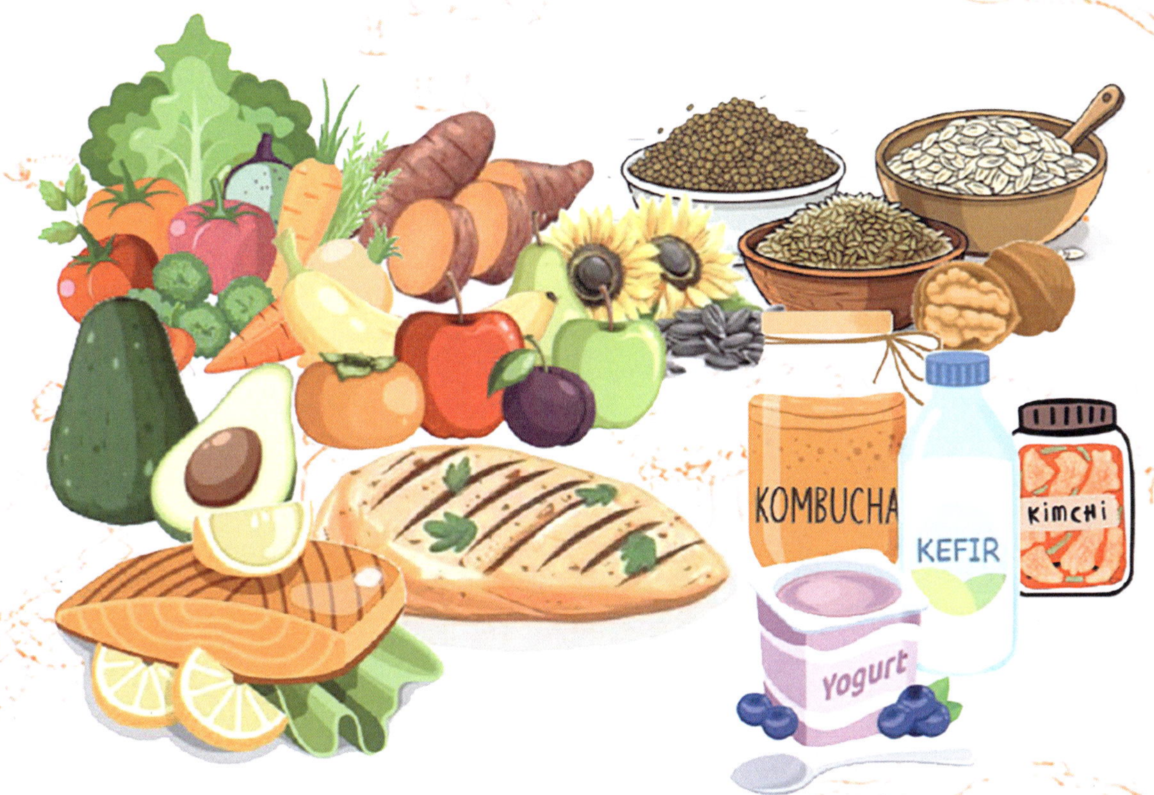

Also, the skin of people with eczema has a hard time keeping
moisture inside the body. That means you can become
dehydrated more easily, especially when your disease is
flaring. So make sure to drink lots of water!

When reading about dietary advice, keep in mind that the term "processed food" can mean something different to a scientist working on research than it does to a typical customer at the grocery store. Current definitions of processed foods, or ultra-processed foods, are often focused on the steps it takes to make something. So, breads may all be labeled "ultra-processed" because of the effort needed to go from a stalk of wheat in the field to a loaf on the table. Obviously, some breads contain preservatives and added sugars, and some do not, so painting all as bad (or defending all as good because of a shaky definition) is not scientifically sound. Current research is trying to sort out if the harm associated with some foods is due to the processing itself or the ingredients that are typically found in foods that require processing. We suspect that it will be the ingredients that are the issue, but people should be aware that reading about "ultra-processed diets" can be tricky due to variable definitions.

One other note: Please talk to your provider before completely eliminating any food from your diet. Patients and caregivers often report that specific foods worsen their eczema - with milk dairy being the most common suspect. However, doctors typically think of food allergies in terms of severe reactions like anaphylaxis (where people's face or tongue swell, they have trouble breathing, and their blood pressure drops). Since the tests for food allergies are built for anaphylaxis, they are often negative even when a patient is certain their eczema reacts to specific foods. But, while avoiding the foods might help your eczema, there is a risk that doing so will cause your reaction to go from eczema-worsening to anaphylaxis (32, 34).

It is a very complicated balance to try to keep. Thus, you
should talk to an allergist about any specific food concerns
and get recommendations on how to keep small amounts in your
diet - small-enough amounts that they won't worsen your skin,
but enough to protect against developing anaphylaxic
reactions. Your allergist may also want to test your blood
for signs of severe allergies (called an IgE test).

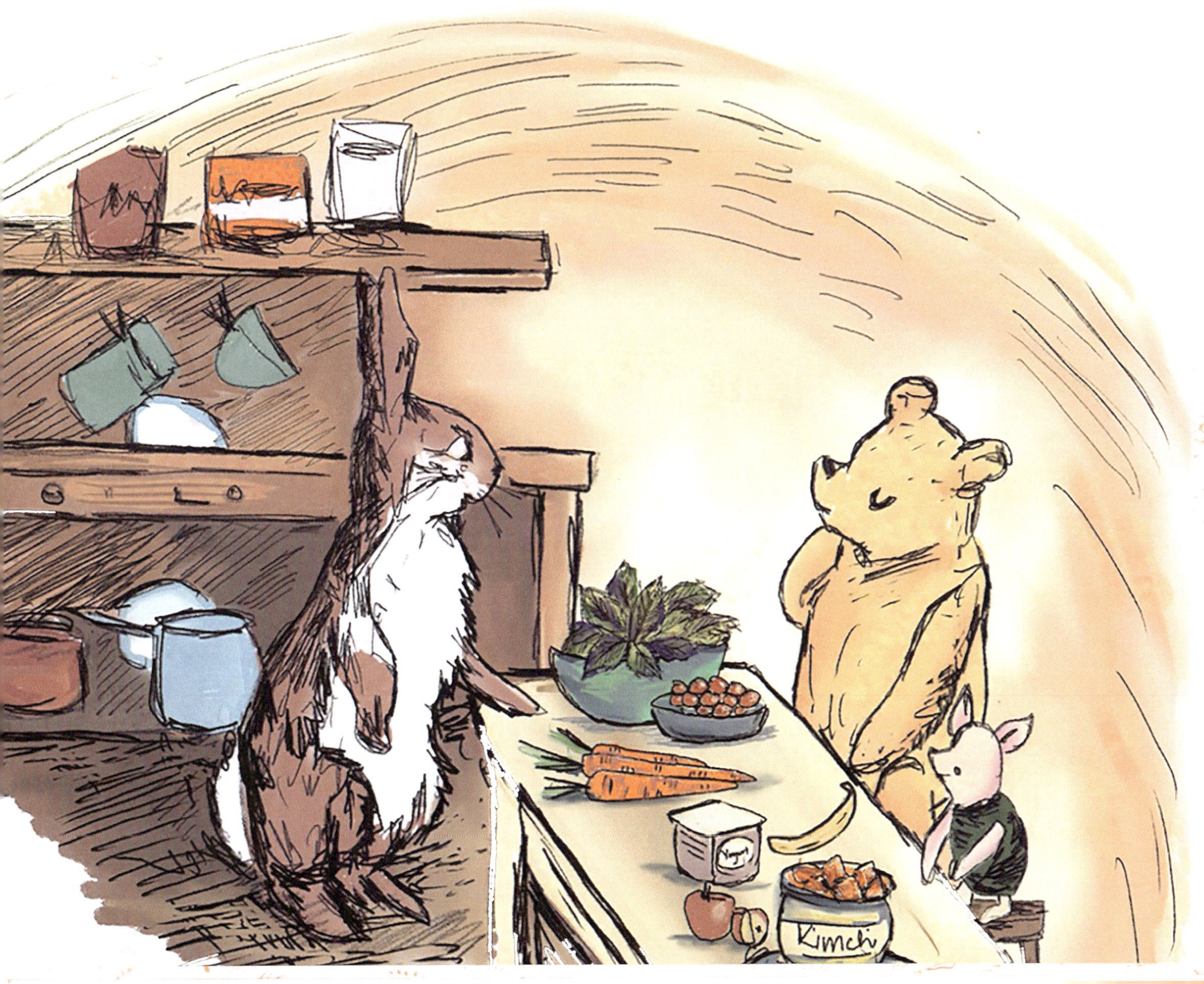

Bathing advice

Most parents and patients already know the advice about bathing in lukewarm water (not hot water, since that can cause more blood and inflammation to come into the skin)(35). Usually soaking for at least 10-15 minutes, three times per week, is recommended. However, there is no evidence that either the timing (morning or evening) or duration of bathing matters (36). When you are done bathing, you should blot dry instead of wiping, since wiping is more abrasive.

It is important to know that when it comes to bathing and washing, water alone can be enough. Soaps are, by definition, substances that disrupt what are known as "lipid membranes" – a protective layer for your skin (37-38). Think about a greasy pan or dish. Trying to clean with just water causes the grease to simply smear around the pan. But when you use soap, the grease comes off. That is because the bonds between different molecules of grease are being broken by the soap. The soap stops the grease from sticking together as a smear and allows it to be washed away. When it comes to cleaning off grease, this is very helpful. However, your skin is (more or less) one giant lipid membrane. While there are proteins and other things in the skin, it functions as a lipid membrane. So, using soap when it isn't needed can disrupt the skin's natural lipid membranes and get in the way of the skin's ability to do the job of protecting our bodies from the outside world.

Soaps also can contain preservatives or other ingredients that kill microorganisms. This can be a great thing when we remove harmful bacteria from our hands. However, using it unnecessarily might risk killing the microbiome of the skin (39).

The microbiome of the skin includes the bacteria that are
supposed to live on our skin and help our skin stay
healthy. So, please use soap when you are worried about
infections, when you need to wash your hands after using
the bathroom, or when you or your child is soiled. But
there is no need to use soap routinely, especially for
infants. Once again, the apps and websites mentioned
before can help inform parents and patients about
whether the soap they are buying contains chemicals of
concern. When soap is used, the mildest version is
preferred.

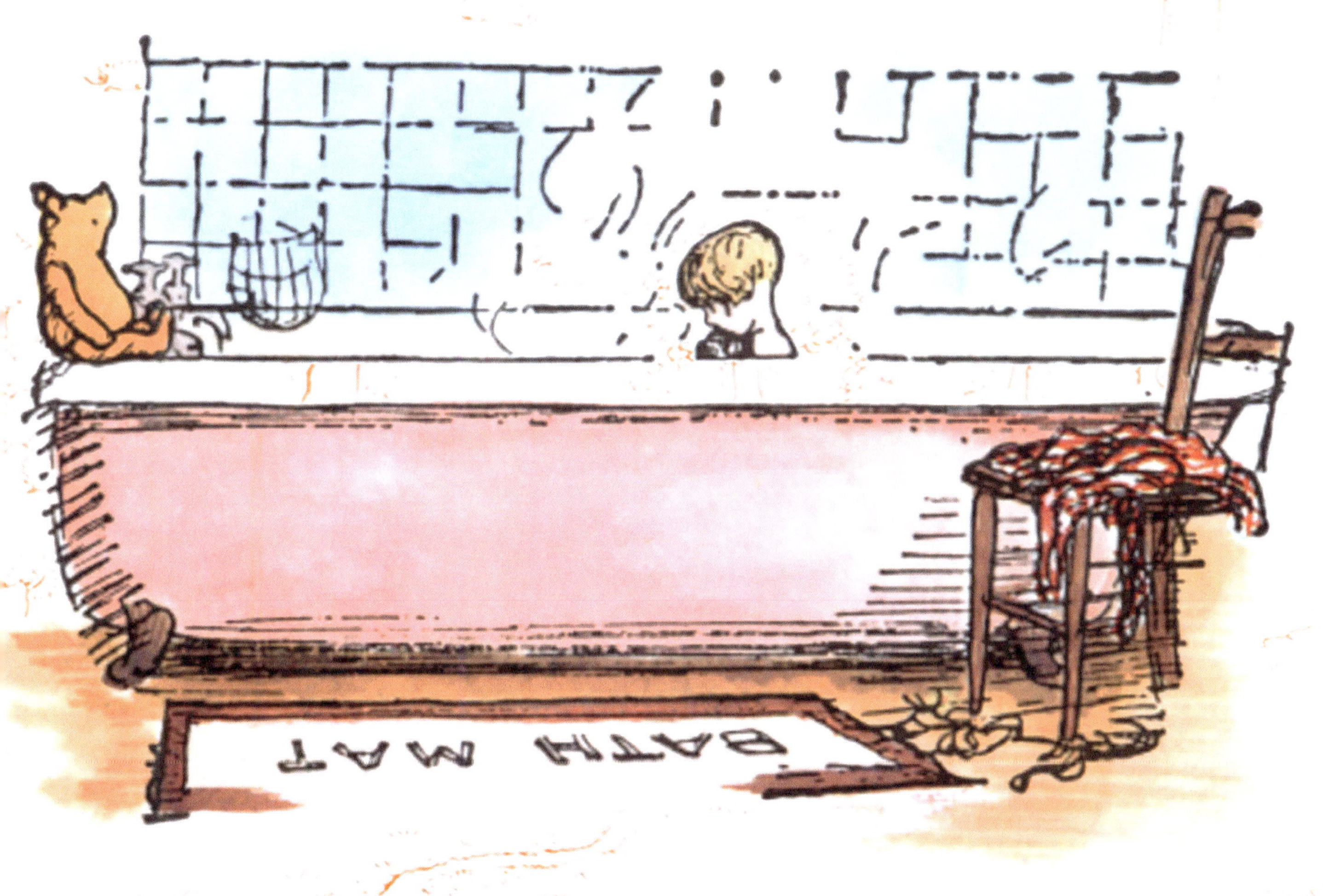

Moisturizers

There are lots of different options for moisturizers out there. It is difficult to tell anyone a specific one to use. However, the evidence suggests that moisturizers that are lipid-based and contain ceramides improve symptoms of eczema better than moisturizers that do not have these ingredients (40-41). Keep in mind that "ceramides" is a category of lipids. That means that two different products might contain completely different types of ceramides. Until research is done to establish which specific types of ceramides are best for skin products, trial and error is sadly the only option for patients and caregivers.

Be wary of moisturizers that contain alcohols. Some alcohols are okay, especially for people with completely healthy skin. However, if you read the ingredients and see a lot of different types of alcohols, or if "alcohol" is one of the first few ingredients listed, there is a risk that the product will cause burning in patients with eczema. We can also firmly say that you should never use any moisturizers that come in a tub that you would need to put your hands in to scoop out the product. This is true even if you use a spoon or something else to remove the moisturizer (and avoid putting your hands directly into the tub). In order to prevent bacteria from your hands from contaminating their product in the tub, companies add more bacteria-killing ingredients. Many of those ingredients kill the healthy bacteria on your skin as well. There are far too many products to test for the impact on the skin's microbiome, but we have found that the following do not seem to cause harm:

Atopalm MLE Cream, Aveeno Colloidal Oatmeal, CeraVe Daily
Moisturizing Lotion, Cetaphil Moisturizing Cream, Codex Eczema
Relief Lotion, Eczema Honey Lotion, Eucerin Original Healing
Lotion, RareGlo Skin & Hair Butter, Simple Sugars Coconut Body
Lotion, Vanicream Lotion, CeraVe Healing Ointment, Vaseline
Advanced Repair Lotion, Dr Bronner's Coconut Oil, Codex Eczema
Relief Lotion, Kiyamel Eczema Relief Oil, Nutiva Liquid Coconut
Oil, Spectrum Culinary Sunflower Oil, and Neutrogena Sheer Zinc
Sunscreen.

However, the following products are harmful to the skin's
normal bacteria, and we recommend avoiding them: Aveeno Eczema
Therapy, Curel HydraTherapy, Eucerin Eczema Relief Cream,
Lubriderm Daily Moisture Lotion, Aquaphor Healing Ointment,
Spectrum Culinary Canola Oil, Spectrum Culinary Grapeseed Oil,
Spectrum Culinary Olive Oil, Banana Boat Sport Ultra Sunscreen
Spray, Neutrogena Beach Defense Sunscreen Spray, and Coppertone
Sport Sunscreen Spray

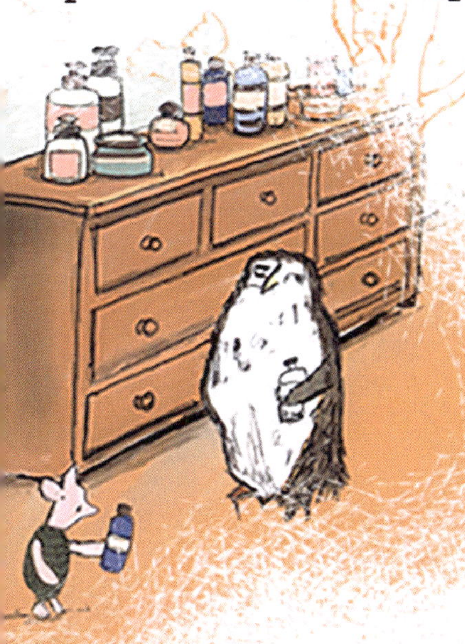

In the United States, the law states
that companies can put the word "eczema"
on the label of their skin care product
if it has above a specified amount of
either colloidal oatmeal or mineral oil
(42). That is all that is required.
So, if you see a product marked as "for
eczema," all you know is that it
contains one or both of those
ingredients. Colloidal oatmeal and
mineral oil are not harmful, but the
benefit from using them is small, if
anything.

Probiotics

Think of probiotics as a way to replant a garden. Planting seeds does not help right away, but once the beneficial plants have grown, they can continue to help even if you stop seeding. But also like a garden, the results take time. It takes several weeks to see benefits from using probiotics (either topically or as pills), so don't give up if you don't see results right away.

Probiotics may help eczema, but there is a lot of complexity (and confusion!) about which specific probiotics help. Every probiotic contains different organisms, which have their own unique chemistry and actions.

This makes comparing probiotics difficult. One firm piece of advice is that probiotics worth considering should list the genus, species, and strain identifiers. Typically, that would be written as something like "*Genus species* ABC1234" or "*G. species* ABC1234". The only exception is LGG, which is an abbreviation for the strain *L. rhamnosus* GG. Any probiotic that does not have that level of detail (such as saying only "*Lactobacillus*" or "*B. fragilus*" without any strain number) is less likely to be legitimate and should be avoided (43-45).

Our research group works on a topical probiotic called *Roseomonas mucosa* RSM2015 (46-52). It can be found over the counter under the name Defensin, sold by the company Skinesa. In full disclosure, our employer (the National Institutes of Health) has a licensing agreement with Skinesa, so we each have a conflict of interest there. While we continue to research *R. mucosa* RSM2015, we have thus far found it can help reduce itching and rashes due to eczema. Probiotics like RSM2015 also have the advantage of being able to live on the skin after you have finished treatment. So you might only need to treat the skin for a few months; then the bacteria will continue to live there and produce healthy fats for your skin even if you stop treatment.

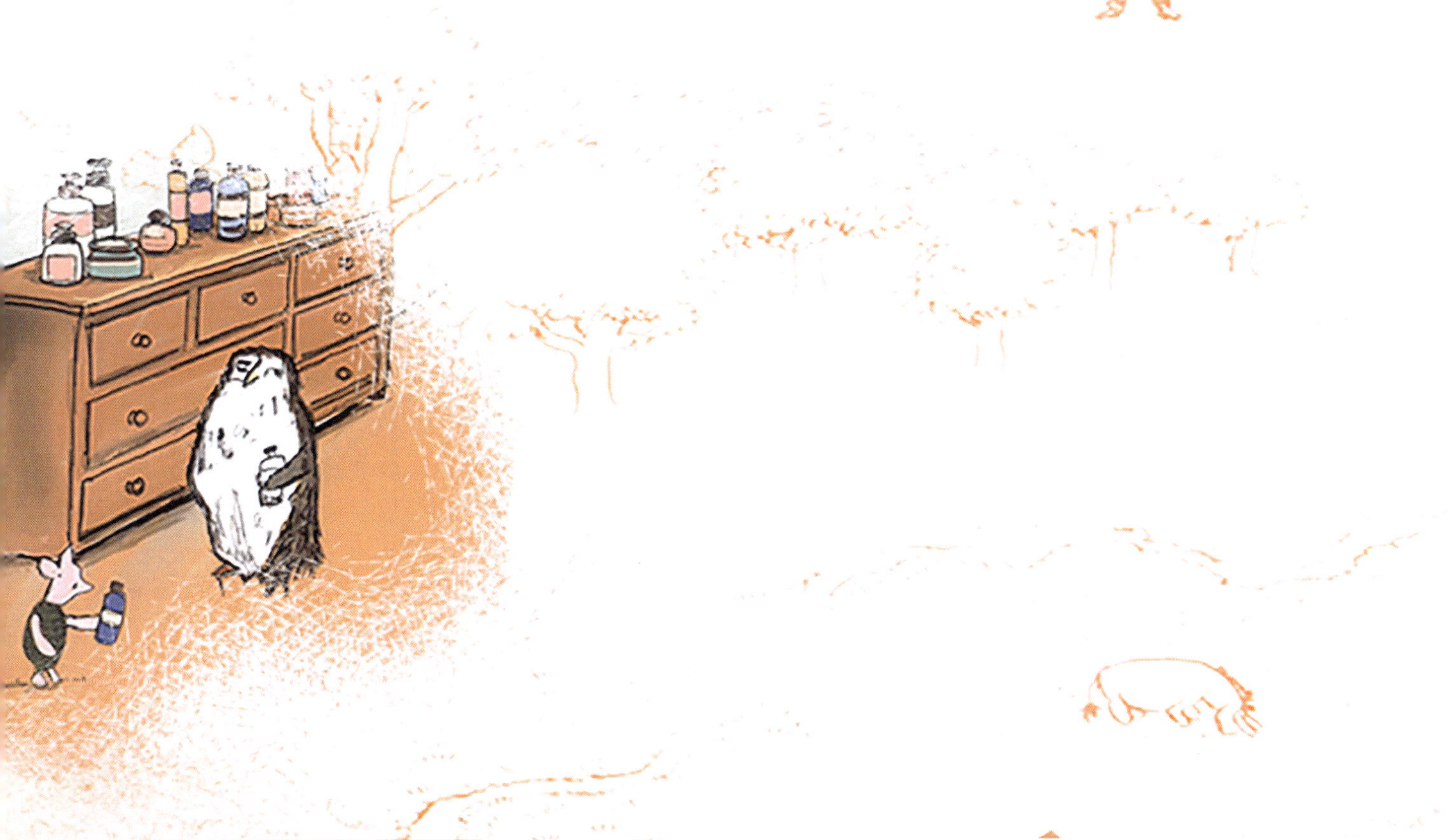

Getting social and emotional support

Eczema is a very taxing disorder - physically and emotionally (53-56). Even when the skin is under good control, the constant need for treatments and worry about flares can take an emotional toll. When the skin is not under good control, the constant itch and poor sleep can be a major stressor for both patients and caregivers. It is important to admit that dealing with eczema is hard (57). It is not "just a rash."

There are groups that can provide some emotional support as well as a community to share ideas and experiences with. For example, the National Eczema Association (NEA) offers toll-free counseling at 1-800-818-7546, but this is limited to the USA during normal business hours. Global Parents for Eczema Research (GPER) runs a support program for eczema caregivers, which can be found at www.gper.org/caregiver.

Having emotional support and mental health check-ins is especially important for teens and young adults who must deal with the disease and the social isolation that comes with it.

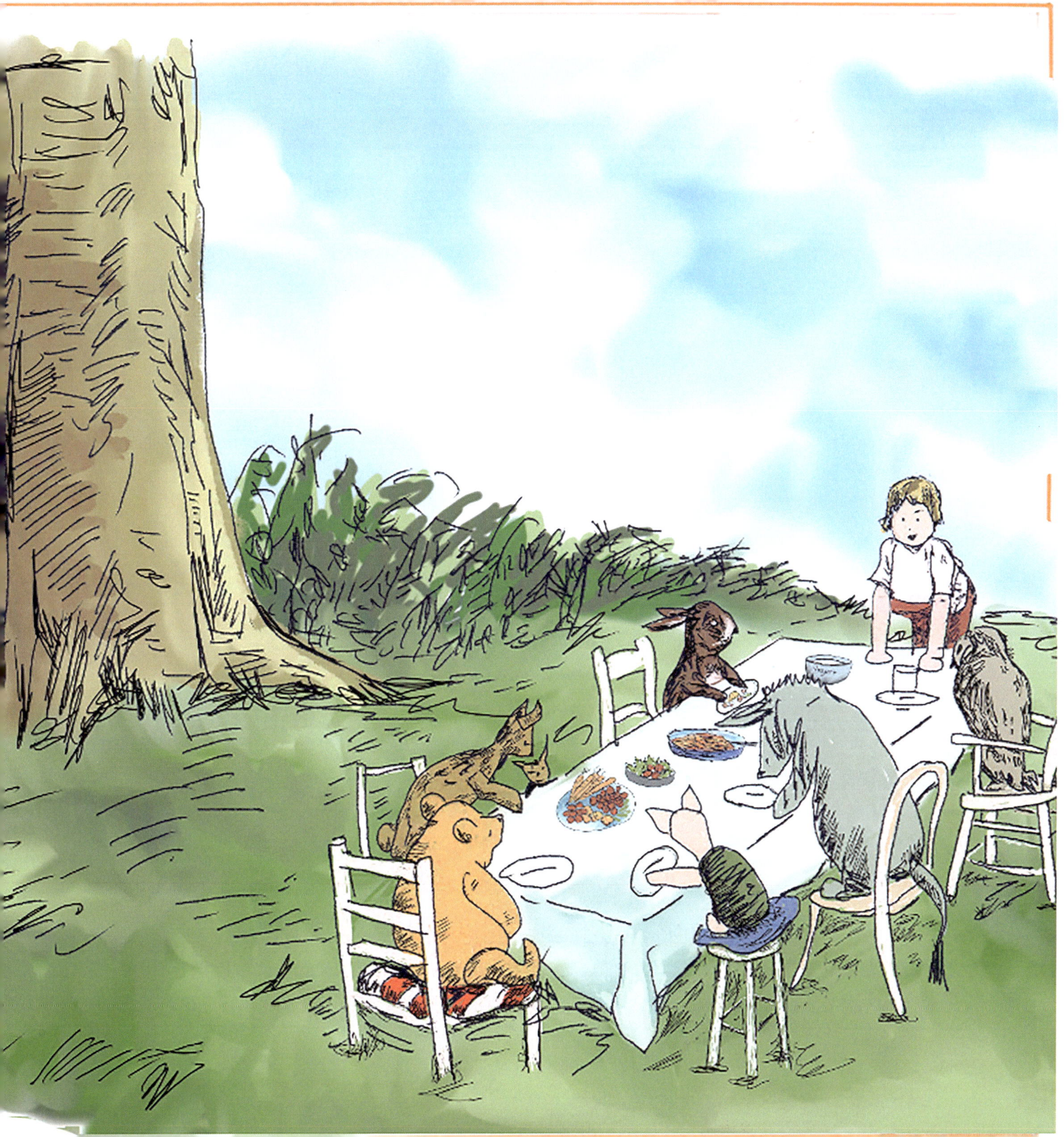

Limitations

A major limitation of our suggestions is that they are mostly extrapolations. For example, we might know that specific chemicals are linked to eczema by time and location, meaning that places and eras with more of those chemicals tend to have more eczema sufferers. We may observe that products containing those chemicals tend to flare people's eczema. We might also know that those chemicals cause eczema in mice or create other harms related to eczema, like disrupting the microbiome. However, that does not ensure that avoiding those chemicals in someone who already has the disease will improve disease control. However, there is more than enough evidence to make our suggestions, especially since there is no reason to suspect that any of them would be harmful.

Still, more research is needed. Research groups, including ours, are currently conducting research to establish how much benefit is possible through avoiding triggers. Hypothetically, one day we might discover that air purification is more important while bedsheet material is not. So this is the best picture we have right now, but future evidence may provide further clarity.

Taking broader action

Finally, for those who want to consider taking broader action for eczema, consider reaching out to the eczema advocacy groups like GPER, NEA, or AAFA.

You could also push for rules that require companies to put warning labels on products that contain eczema-worsening chemicals. Furthermore - and if we are being completely honest - there needs to be collective action against the unquestioned use of these chemicals in our environments.

While the average person can control what products they
bring into their home, they cannot control the amount of
chemicals released from nearby factories or highways.
Fixing that issue is much larger than what one silly ol'
bear could tackle. But it is something we need to think
about if we want to clean up all of our woods.

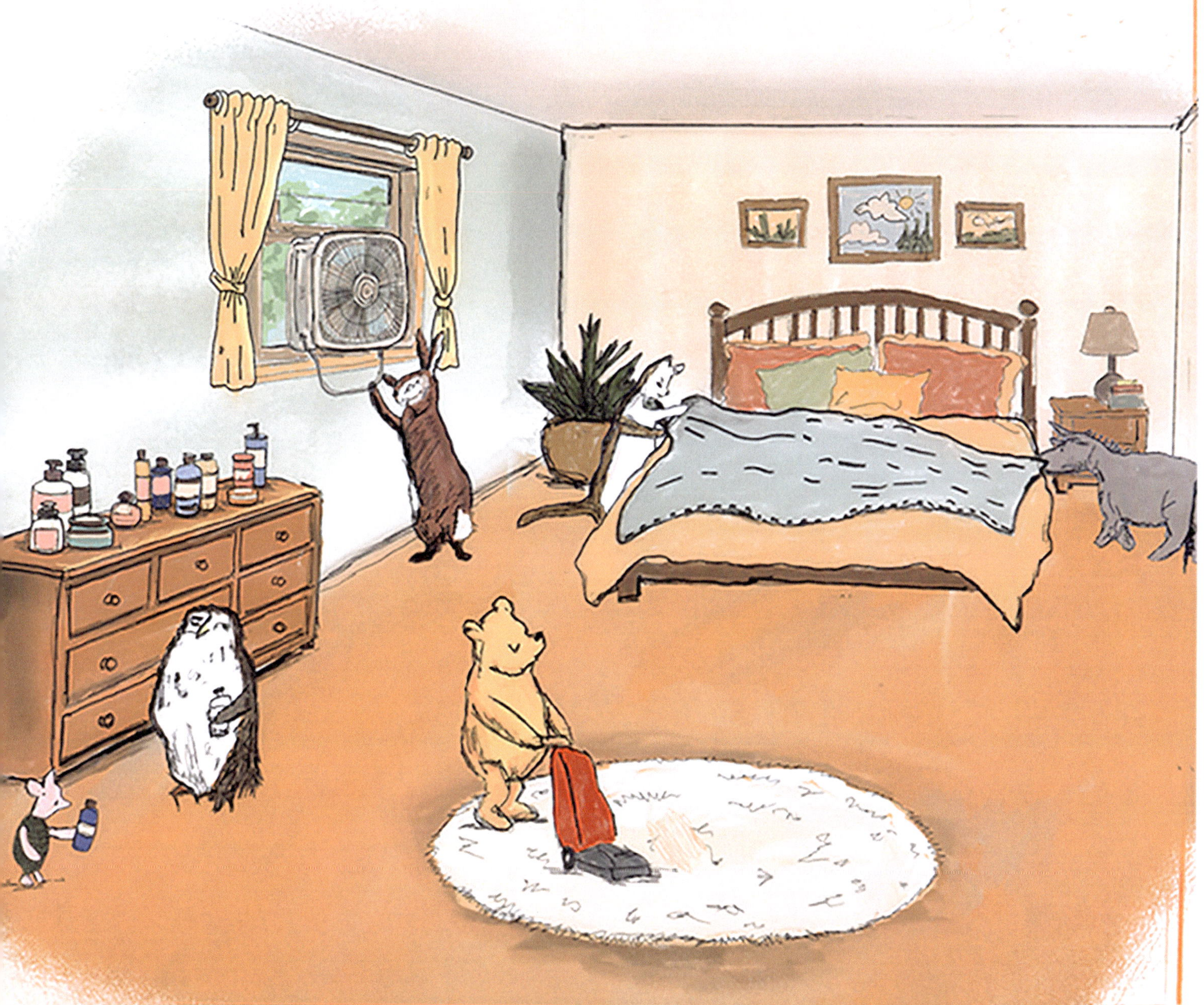

References

1. Yuka. Make the right choices for your health. (Yuka.io/en/).
2. EWG. EWG's Healthy Living App. (https://www.ewg.org).
3. SkinSafe. Vol. 2024 (2024).
4. Ng, Y.T. & Chew, F.T. A systematic review and meta-analysis of risk factors associated with atopic dermatitis in Asia. World Allergy Organ J 13, 100477 (2020).
5. Herbarth, O., et al. Association between indoor renovation activities and eczema in early childhood. Int J Hyg Environ Health 209, 241-247 (2006).
6. Lee, J.H., et al. Surveillance of home environment in children with atopic dermatitis: a questionnaire survey. Asia Pac Allergy 2, 59-66 (2012).
7. Rinaldi, A.O., et al. Household laundry detergents disrupt barrier integrity and induce inflammation in mouse and human skin. Allergy 79, 128-141 (2024).
8. Akdis, C.A. Does the epithelial barrier hypothesis explain the increase in allergy, autoimmunity and other chronic conditions? Nat Rev Immunol 21, 739-751 (2021).
9. von Holst, H., et al. Perfluoroalkyl substances exposure and immunity, allergic response, infection, and asthma in children: review of epidemiologic studies. Heliyon 7, e08160 (2021).
10. Calderon, L., et al. Air concentrations of volatile organic compounds associated with conventional and "green" cleaning products in real-world and laboratory settings. Indoor Air 32, e13162 (2022).
11. Ogulur, I., et al. Gut epithelial barrier damage caused by dishwasher detergents and rinse aids. J Allergy Clin Immunol 151, 469-484 (2023).
12. Langan, S.M., Silcocks, P. & Williams, H.C. What causes flares of eczema in children? Br J Dermatol 161, 640-646 (2009).
13. Mason, R. Fabrics for atopic dermatitis. J Fam Health Care 18, 63-65 (2008).
14. Shen, D., et al. Evaluation of Polycyclic Aromatic Hydrocarbons (PAHs) in Bamboo Shoots from Soil. Bull Environ Contam Toxicol 106, 589-593 (2021).
15. Bian, F., Zhong, Z., Zhang, X., Yang, C. & Gai, X. Bamboo - An untapped plant resource for the phytoremediation of heavy metal contaminated soils. Chemosphere 246, 125750 (2020).
16. Bolden, A.L., Kwiatkowski, C.F. & Colborn, T. New Look at BTEX: Are Ambient Levels a Problem? Environ Sci Technol 49, 5261-5276 (2015).
17. Registry), A.A.f.T.S.a.D. Medical Management Guidelines for Toluene Diisocyanate. (Cdc.gov).
18. Kim, Y.M., Kim, J., Ha, S.C. & Ahn, K. Effects of Exposure to Indoor Fine Particulate Matter on Atopic Dermatitis in Children. Int J Environ Res Public Health 18(2021).
19. Azimi, P. & Stephens, B. A framework for estimating the US mortality burden of fine particulate matter exposure attributable to indoor and outdoor microenvironments. J Expo Sci Environ Epidemiol 30, 271-284 (2020).
20. Messier, K.P., et al. Indoor versus Outdoor Air Quality during Wildfires. Environ Sci Technol Lett 6, 696-701 (2019).
21. Walker, E.S., Stewart, T. & Jones, D. Fine particulate matter infiltration at Western Montana residences during wildfire season. Sci Total Environ 896, 165238 (2023).
22. Li, J., et al. The persistence of smoke VOCs indoors: Partitioning, surface cleaning, and air cleaning in a smoke-contaminated house. Sci Adv 9, eadh8263 (2023).

23. Sriprapat, W., Boraphech, P. & Thiravetyan, P. Factors affecting xylene-contaminated air removal by the ornamental plant Zamioculcas zamiifolia. Environ Sci Pollut Res Int 21, 2603-2610 (2014).

24. Kim, K.J., et al. Removal ratio of gaseous toluene and xylene transported from air to root zone via the stem by indoor plants. Environ Sci Pollut Res Int 23, 6149-6158 (2016).

25. Matheson, S., Fleck, R., Irga, P.J. & Torpy, F.R. Phytoremediation for the indoor environment: a state-of-the-art review. Rev Environ Sci Biotechnol 22, 249-280 (2023).

26. Kumar, R., Verma, V., Thakur, M., Singh, G. & Bhargava, B. A systematic review on mitigation of common indoor air pollutants using plant-based methods: a phytoremediation approach. Air Qual Atmos Health, 1-27 (2023).

27. Tan, T., et al. Maternal yogurt consumption during pregnancy and infantile eczema: a prospective cohort study. Food Funct 14, 1929-1936 (2023).

28. Kim, H.J., Ju, S.Y. & Park, Y.K. Kimchi intake and atopic dermatitis in Korean aged 19-49 years: The Korea National Health and Nutrition Examination Survey 2010-2012. Asia Pac J Clin Nutr 26, 914-922 (2017).

29. Venter, C., et al. The maternal diet index in pregnancy is associated with offspring allergic diseases: the Healthy Start study. Allergy 77, 162-172 (2022).

30. Park, S. & Bae, J.H. Fermented food intake is associated with a reduced likelihood of atopic dermatitis in an adult population (Korean National Health and Nutrition Examination Survey 2012-2013). Nutr Res 36, 125-133 (2016).

31. Ercelik, H.C. & Kaya, V. The effects of fermented food consumption in pregnancy on neonatal and infant health: An integrative review. J Pediatr Nurs 75, 173-179 (2023).

32. Khan, A., Adalsteinsson, J. & Whitaker-Worth, D.L. Atopic dermatitis and nutrition. Clin Dermatol 40, 135-144 (2022).

33. Venter, C. Immunonutrition: Diet Diversity, Gut Microbiome and Prevention of Allergic Diseases. Allergy Asthma Immunol Res 15, 545-561 (2023).

34. Oykhman, P., et al. Dietary Elimination for the Treatment of Atopic Dermatitis: A Systematic Review and Meta-Analysis. J Allergy Clin Immunol Pract 10, 2657-2666 e2658 (2022).

35. Cardona, I.D., Kempe, E.E., Lary, C., Ginder, J.H. & Jain, N. Frequent Versus Infrequent Bathing in Pediatric Atopic Dermatitis: A Randomized Clinical Trial. J Allergy Clin Immunol Pract 8, 1014-1021 (2020).

36. Allan, G.M., Craig, R. & Korownyk, C.S. Atopic dermatitis and bathing. Can Fam Physician 67, 758 (2021).

37. Henriksen, J.R., Andresen, T.L., Feldborg, L.N., Duelund, L. & Ipsen, J.H. Understanding detergent effects on lipid membranes: a model study of lysolipids. Biophys J 98, 2199-2205 (2010).

38. Mijaljica, D., Spada, F. & Harrison, I.P. Skin Cleansing without or with Compromise: Soaps and Syndets. Molecules 27 (2022).

39. Gough, P., Khalid, M.B., Hartono, S. & Myles, I.A. Microbial manipulation in atopic dermatitis. Clin Transl Med 12, e828 (2022).

40. Sindher, S., et al. Pilot study measuring transepidermal water loss (TEWL) in children suggests trilipid cream is more effective than a paraffin-based emollient. Allergy 75, 2662-2664 (2020).

41. Elias, P.M. Optimizing emollient therapy for skin barrier repair in atopic dermatitis. Ann Allergy Asthma Immunol 128, 505-511 (2022).

42. Shobnam, N., Ratley, G., Zeldin, J., Yadav, M. & Myles, I.A. Environmental and behavioral mitigation strategies for patients with atopic dermatitis. JAAD Int 17, 181-191 (2024).

43. Xue, X., Yang, X., Shi, X. & Deng, Z. Efficacy of probiotics in pediatric atopic dermatitis: A systematic review and meta-analysis. Clin Transl Allergy 13, e12283 (2023).

44. Makrgeorgou, A., et al. Probiotics for treating eczema. Cochrane Database Syst Rev 11, CD006135 (2018).

45. Tan-Lim, C.S.C., et al. Comparative effectiveness of probiotic strains on the prevention of pediatric atopic dermatitis: A systematic review and network meta-analysis. Pediatr Allergy Immunol 32, 1255-1270 (2021).

46. Myles, I.A., Moore, I.N., Castillo, C.R. & Datta, S.K. Differing Virulence of Healthy Skin Commensals in Mouse Models of Infection. Front Cell Infect Microbiol 8, 451 (2018).

47. Myles, I.A., et al. Transplantation of human skin microbiota in models of atopic dermatitis. JCI Insight 1(2016).

48. Myles, I.A., et al. A method for culturing Gram-negative skin microbiota. BMC Microbiol 16, 60 (2016).

49. Jacobson, M.E., Myles, I.A., Paller, A.S., Eichenfield, L.F. & Simpson, E.L. A Randomized, Double-Blind, Placebo-Controlled, Multicenter, 16-Week Trial to Evaluate the Efficacy and Safety of FB-401 in Children, Adolescents, and Adult Subjects (Ages 2 Years and Older) with Mild-to-Moderate Atopic Dermatitis. Dermatology 240, 85-94 (2024).

50. Zeldin, J., et al. Exposure to isocyanates predicts atopic dermatitis prevalence and disrupts therapeutic pathways in commensal bacteria. Sci Adv 9, eade8898 (2023).

51. Myles, I.A., et al. First-in-human topical microbiome transplantation with Roseomonas mucosa for atopic dermatitis. JCI Insight 3(2018).

52. Myles, I.A., et al. Therapeutic responses to Roseomonas mucosa in atopic dermatitis may involve lipid-mediated TNF-related epithelial repair. Sci Transl Med 12(2020).

53. Panel, A.A.J.A.D.G., et al. Atopic dermatitis (eczema) guidelines: 2023 American Academy of Allergy, Asthma and Immunology/American College of Allergy, Asthma and Immunology Joint Task Force on Practice Parameters GRADE- and Institute of Medicine-based recommendations. Ann Allergy Asthma Immunol (2023).

54. Cai, X.C., et al. Epidemiology of mental health comorbidity in patients with atopic dermatitis: An analysis of global trends from 1998 to 2022. J Eur Acad Dermatol Venereol 38, 496-512 (2024).

55. Sandhu, J.K., Wu, K.K., Bui, T.L. & Armstrong, A.W. Association Between Atopic Dermatitis and Suicidality: A Systematic Review and Meta-analysis. JAMA Dermatol 155, 178-187 (2019).

56. Kelly, K.A., Balogh, E.A., Kaplan, S.G. & Feldman, S.R. Skin Disease in Children: Effects on Quality of Life, Stigmatization, Bullying, and Suicide Risk in Pediatric Acne, Atopic Dermatitis, and Psoriasis Patients. Children (Basel) 8(2021).

57. Radtke, S., Grossberg, A.L. & Wan, J. Mental health comorbidity in youth with atopic dermatitis: A narrative review of possible mechanisms. Pediatr Dermatol 40, 977-982 (2023).

ABOUT THE AUTHORS

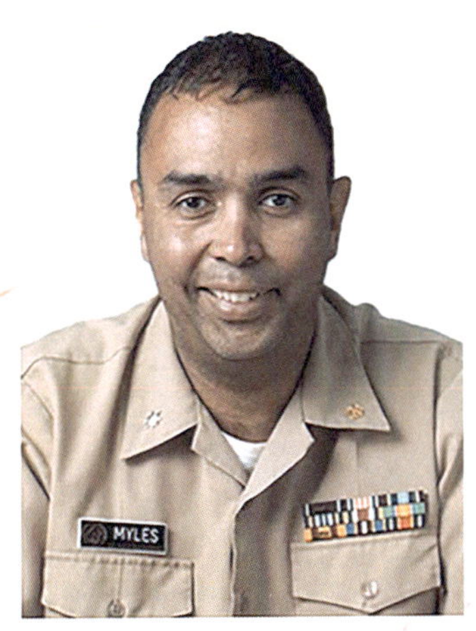

Ian A. Myles, MD/MPH. Dr. Myles grew up in Colorado. After medical school he trained in internal medicine before training in allergy and clinical immunology. He has worked as a researcher for over 15 years, investigating how environmental factors impact allergic disease. He has authored more than 80 peer-reviewed publications on eczema, allergies, and topical steroid withdrawal. Dr. Myles has also authored a book, GATTACA Has Fallen, which is about the harms of researchers looking for the "gene for" common diseases like eczema at the expense of researching environmental causes. His research lab has partnered with numerous patient advocacy groups over the years. Overall, his work has educated the public on the environmental causes of allergic disease and produced the first topical probiotic targeted for eczema treatment. He continues to serve as the chief of The Epithelial Therapeutics Unit and as a medical officer in the United States uniformed service.

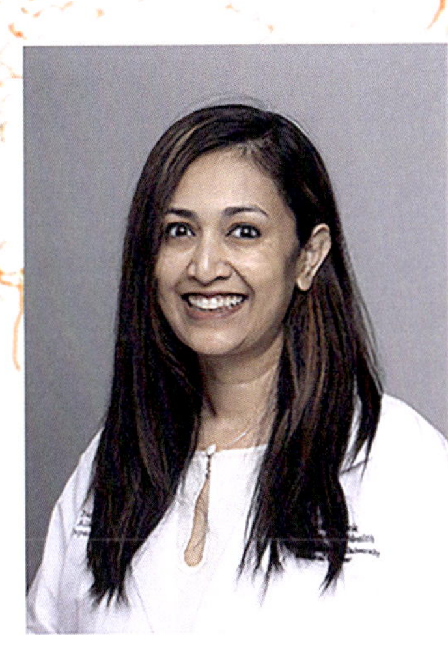

Nadia Bhandari (Shobnam), MD. Dr. Bhandari grew up in Delaware. After medical school, she trained in pediatrics before specializing in allergy and immunology. She is currently a practicing allergist and immunologist with a focus on dermatologic and allergic conditions. She has a specific focus on eczema and environmental contributors to atopic disease. She has hands-on clinical experience caring for patients with eczema and has authored several peer-reviewed publications on atopic dermatitis and other skin diseases. Through her clinical work and writing, Dr. Bhandari is dedicated to translating evidence-based medicine into practical, accessible guidance for patients and families.